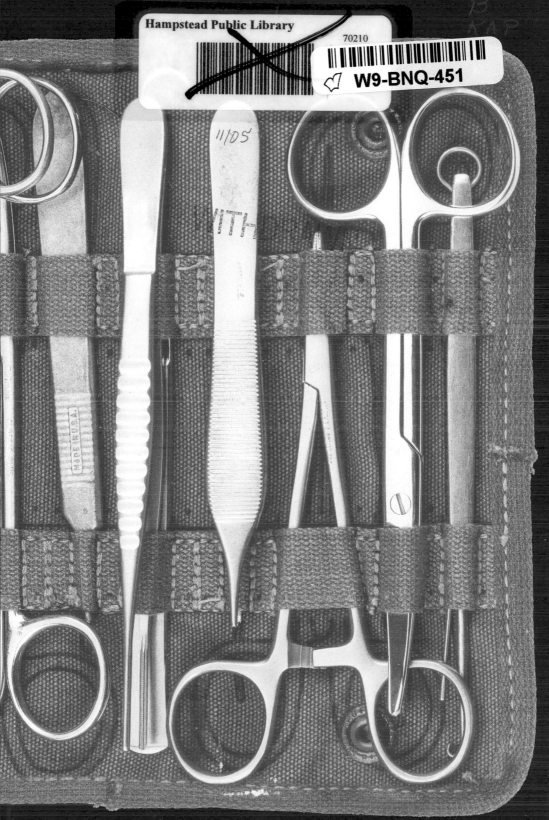

Hampstead Public Library

Contact Wounds

ALSO BY THE AUTHOR

The Dressing Station

Jonathan Kaplan

Contact Wounds

A War Surgeon's Education

HAMPSTEAD PUBLIC LIBRARY
P.O. BOX 190
HAMPSTEAD, NH 03841

Grove Press
New York

Copyright © 2005 by Jonathan Kaplan

All rights reserved. No part of this book may be reproduced in any form
or by any electronic or mechanical means, including information storage and
retrieval systems, without permission in writing from the publisher, except by a
reviewer, who may quote brief passages in a review. Any members of educational
institutions wishing to photocopy part or all of the work for classroom use, or
publishers who would like to obtain permission to include the work in an
anthology, should send their inquiries to Grove/Atlantic, Inc., 841 Broadway,
New York, NY 10003.

Published simultaneously in Canada
Printed in the United States of America

FIRST EDITION

Library of Congress Cataloging-in-Publication Data

Kaplan, Jonathan, 1954–
    Contact wounds : a war surgeon's education / Jonathan Kaplan.
      p. cm.
    ISBN 0-8021-1800-3
    1. Kaplan, Jonathan, 1954-   2. Surgery, Military—Biography.   I. Title.

  RD153.K37 2005
  617'.092—dc22   2005050204
  [B]

Grove Press
an imprint of Grove/Atlantic, Inc.
841 Broadway
New York, NY 10003

05 06 07 08 09   10 9 8 7 6 5 4 3 2 1

For Andrew, Greg, Peter, Jacqui, Neil, Linda, Graeme, Jean, Margaret and all those whose names I didn't know.

Contents

Prodrome
Contact Wounds

Life's passage is peaceful only for the fortunate. For those of us who become surgeons it is a search for sureness, amidst potential missteps and knife-edge decisions. Each of these situations leaves marks – contact wounds – that signpost a physical and emotional journey. This one begins with a colonial childhood, caught between old conflicts and new unrest. It takes in riots, wars, tropical medicine, documentary film-making, forensic investigations, a jungle search for a missing friend and the murderous streets of Baghdad.

The important things cannot be taught in any medical school. Learning to be a war surgeon is a process of stalking and studying the enemy, death, in order that it may be combated. Such a journey is in the nature of all mythical quests, involving obstacles and digressions, the lure of enlightenment and an implacable foe. It is an education in uncertainty and rootlessness, so that our work and our journeying become an attempt to define our place in the world.

Contact Wounds is an account of these travels, the paths taken and the price paid. Those of us who've been there are all wounded more or less, we have all left parts of ourselves behind. Perhaps none of us was intact to begin with. There's the questionable motivation for voluntarily putting oneself in harm's way; less through bravery or altruism than in flight from some greater loss. We search for completeness in the land of the maimed.

Yet there is a simplicity to existence in those extreme places, a sense of purpose, that can be hard to find in everyday life. This book charts that elusive clarity. It is also a testament to family destiny – for the heritage of our past plays itself out through us, moving our hearts and hands – and to survival, my own and that of the people I've tried to save. Finally, perhaps, it is a dream of the possibility of homecoming.

1

Hereditary Conditions

I used to think we were unlucky that we hadn't had a proper War, and looked for its traces all around me. The buildings along the beachfront were graceful blocks of flats, their corners rounded like an old radio. They had names that I've forgotten, but they held a particular charm for me because, as the adults said so casually, they were 'pre-war'; they had seen history. I imagined cocktail parties on those balconies, guests looking up at the sound of bombers overhead. In truth there hadn't been any bombers over Durban, at least none that flew in anger or rained incendiaries on the town below. The anti-aircraft guns on the Bluff did open up one night in 1941 on an empty sky and a house was demolished by a falling shell; a bit of a joke, really.

But the war had left its mark here, in the names scored on the memorial near the city hall, and grey ships loaded with tanks and men had once sat off the harbour mouth, forming convoys against the enemy submarines that might be stalking them against the imperfect beachfront blackout. My parents and their friends used to talk about those times as we sat on the beach, watching the deep-water swimmers out by the shark-nets. Stories about dancing at the Cosmo Club on leave, getting insults from the Afrikaner Studentebond for being in uniform: not the sort of action I was interested in. When I pressed them they would shake their heads.

'It's 1960,' I was told, 'the war's been over for fifteen years. You don't have to worry about that stuff anymore. Let's have some peace and quiet.'

So I kept quiet and read my war books and tried to make sense of what was going on in the newspapers. The pictures showed police in their flat caps bending over untidy shapes of clothing. The faces were turned away, but I recognised those shapes from pictures of other battlefields. I read the headlines and tried the name 'Sharpeville' on my tongue. It didn't have the same ring as Normandy or Dunkirk, but it meant something to the adults, that was certain, as they sat on the veranda and talked and smoked through the hot evening.

'There's going to be trouble, fighting,' someone said, and I shivered, imagining rubble and tanks rolling through the streets. In the morning as we were being driven to school I stuck my head out of the car window, scanning the sky for aircraft. The other kids sang along with the radio:

'Weatherman
tell us
– *da-dang* –
what's new,
what is the weather going to do?'

There was nothing to see but the morning sun, bouncing off the bay's calm.

It was only when my mother took us shopping in town, the sky black over the buildings before the afternoon thunderstorm, that I began to notice. Lots more cops than usual, elbowing back the unfamiliar weight of their slung rifles. The black people on the streets looked different too: quiet, and walking close to the walls as if they didn't want to attract attention. The police stopped them, lined them up and held out their hands for passbooks. It had a familiar look, like a scene from a movie about the German occupation in France. At the same time I was unimpressed because the cops didn't look like real soldiers and their voices cracked as they shouted.

'*Kom, kaffir*,' they screamed. '*Wys jou pas!*' and I realised how tense they were.

'It's because there's trouble in the Native locations,' I was told by my friend Rolie. 'It's because the Zulus hate the Indians; always have.'

He and his mates suddenly appeared much better informed than I, who only heard evening talk that I wasn't supposed to be listening to, about vague things like 'the political situation'. My school-friends didn't know anything about the political situation – probably didn't know there was one – but they knew about rampages and massacres, had heard their parents talk about black servants who crept silently up the stairs of the white homes each night, carving knife in hand, to check that everyone was asleep.

'My father told me all about it,' said Rolie. 'He was there in '49 during the riots when they burnt the Indian shops. He was called up from the reserves, and they gave him six bullets and a rifle and put him on patrol in Umgeni Road. He said it was the women, the Native women, who stirred it all up, running in front with sticks, making that noise with their tongues. It's just a matter of time before they turn on us.'

And so they went on, comparing rumours, boasting about the size of their fathers' guns, while I listened, perplexed, wondering whether I lived in another country. There was no talk of rifles or homicidal servants at our dinner table, hardly any talk at all that I could follow, but in the evenings the murmur of voices would rise from the terrace below my bedroom, over the sound of trains shunting down at the docks. I leaned on the veranda rail watching the cigarettes glow: Mike and Shirley, Rose and Louie, all those young couples, ice tinkling in their glasses, asking my father about England where he'd been demobilised from the army after the end of the war.

'Oh, it's not so bad there, you know.'

'I couldn't bear it, too cold...' and the women would stand watching the moon rise over the bay with the pressure of that thick, still air on their faces.

✪

The air in Durban had a special embrace, a humidity that held the scent of turmeric and coated your body like honey. Flamingos used to come each year to wade on the mudflats in the bay, near the black whaling ships at anchor with their harpoon-guns shrouded. I imagined it must be very different in Europe, which was the setting of the war books that filled the Adventure section of my local library. I read them late into the night while outside the rainy-season downpour drummed on the giant leaves of the elephant-ear plants and awoke the belling of the tree-frogs. The books were generally about English heroes. I met one once, a legendary World War Two fighter pilot whose biography I'd read over and over. He had lost his legs in a peacetime training crash and was being rehabilitated on metal limbs when the war began. Convincing the Royal Air Force to let him fly again, he led a Group of fighter squadrons against the Germans. He was shot down over France, leaving one of his tin legs behind in the cockpit as he parachuted out, and a spare had to be dropped to him in the camp where he'd been imprisoned. He'd made several attempts to escape, ending the war in the fortress-prison of Colditz. Now the man used his free time to campaign internationally for the care of the disabled; encouraging them, raising money and awareness.

This work brought him to South Africa, to visit the residential handicapped centre in Durban where my father was staff orthopaedic surgeon. I was let off school to meet him. After being shown round and talking to the kids in their wheelchairs, the ex-group-captain sat at a table under the flame lily trees and sucked on his pipe and signed my copy of his book. Back at school my teachers, deeply envious, wanted to know everything about him. They came mostly from England and felt at home in Durban, they said, because this ex-colonial capital on the Indian Ocean reminded them of what Britain had been before standards had declined. Our headmaster had been a prisoner of war – we credited him with many daring, unsuccessful escapes – and wore a tweed jacket and cravat despite the heat. In a locked drawer of his desk he kept a real pistol, which he sometimes showed to groups of deserving boys.

✛

My father had served in the war as a surgeon, treating wounded soldiers in tent field-hospitals. During the desert campaign in North Africa he had watched the barrage flame from horizon to horizon at the battle of El-Alamein, before the arrival of the first ambulances heralded a flood of casualties on which he and his colleagues worked beyond exhaustion. They'd occupied the lulls between battles, or treating wounded from skirmishes and air-raids, with equal application. Among the books in our study was one written by a group of brother medical officers, dated 1943, called *Now There's a Thing: A Manual on the Philosophy and Practice of Liar Dice.* It described lengthy engagements of dare and deception through medical, military and literary allusions, and was extremely funny. Chapters profiled the strategies of maestros of the game; one sketch showed someone who looked like my dad observing a throw through the smoke of his cigarette, dark hair combed back and a captain's pips on the shoulders of his rumpled bush-shirt.

His civilian orthopaedic practice now must have been less intense, but it was often the case that he'd come home from the hospital only after midnight, or be called away during dinner to deal with an emergency. I had a limitless belief in my father's abilities, enhanced by the mysterious kit of clinking bottles he carried in his car-trunk containing powdered plasma, for emergency infusion at the scene of a major accident. His consulting rooms were high in a granite building in downtown Durban, with his name in black on the frosted glass door and a bee-hive-shaped jar of sweets in his desk drawer that my brother and I were allowed to raid when we came to visit. From his window we could look down over the colonial heart of the city; the steps of the old post office where Winston Churchill had addressed the people of Durban after his escape from the Boers in 1900, the city hall flanked by cannons, and the palms around the war memorial with its relief of a mourning angel and the ranks of names. These were all white men's names. The black dead – many had served in the war, as drivers and in labour battalions and other roles that did not involve the carrying of arms – were unlisted. The first story I'd learned of a local war hero, however, was that of Lucas Majozi, a Zulu stretcher-bearer who had gone out under fire at El-Alamein again and again to bring in the wounded despite being wounded repeatedly himself.

It was the war that had taught my father his operating skills. Those years had brought enormous medical advances: in the treatment of shock, in antibiotics, blood transfusion and most significantly in reconstructive surgery, an area in which he'd come to specialise. One afternoon a German lady was brought by a visiting doctor to our house for tea. She'd had her hands blown off when the Hamburg munitions factory in which she had been working had been bombed in 1944. German surgeons had carried out a pioneering reconstructive operation, separating the long bones of her forearms and repositioning tendons so that the muscles performed new movements. Instead of lying together, the bones could now be opened and closed like a crab's claws, allowing her to pick up her cup, place a biscuit between her lips. We sat around the tea table in the garden and I stared aghast as my dad touched those creepy appendages and felt the muscles flex as they pinched.

'That's beautiful,' he said. The German lady was pretty – she'd been a girl when the injury happened – and suddenly I saw her blush.

The orthopaedic work he did for the handicapped centre involved similar reconstructive techniques. Most of the children suffered from muscle spasticity due to cerebral palsy, and my father would perform tendon transfers – he'd explain to me the operations required, pointing out the muscles on my own skinny arms and legs – loosening contractions and shifting the pull of one over-active muscle to counter another so that a limb could be made straight; that's what the Greek word *orthos* meant. He addressed medical conferences on the surgical treatment of spinal tuberculosis, to straighten backs crooked by bone collapse and take pressure off the spinal cord. For the Zulu leprosy patients at the sanatorium up the coast he carried out operations to correct deformities caused by nerve damage from the disease. We always knew when he'd been working there, for – despite his knowledge of leprosy's low infectivity – he would fend off our greetings and step out of his workclothes in the upstairs passage that led from the garage, in order to shower and change before joining us at the dinner table.

My mother usually came home smelling of disinfectant. She was a pathologist, working at the medical school. Pathology was as fascinating as surgery but more solemn, because it was about death. One of the heads of her department was carrying out research into the techniques of suicide favoured by each of the city's ethnic groups. Black men cut their throats. Black women drank bleach. Indian women set themselves alight, the men hanged themselves. White women took overdoses, while the most popular technique for white men – apart from a brief vogue of looping a rope round the neck, tying the other end to a tree, and driving off at speed – was their readily-to-hand firearms.

There were two kinds of white people, English and Afrikaans. The latter spoke a different language; also, while we had been fighting the Germans in World War Two, the Afrikaner opposition party headed by Dr Malan (a Doctor of Divinity, I was relieved to note, not of medicine) had wanted a Nazi victory. Afrikaner students attacked soldiers on leave. My mother had been at Pretoria University at the time, while her brothers were serving in North Africa. She remembered some of her classmates giving the Hitler salute, and the night a sabotage group had derailed a troop train by blowing up the line where it ran through the *veld* near her family home east of the city. Now the Afrikaners ran the country and made the laws, and the political discussions among my parents and their friends involved a certain seriousness of tone that tended to set them beyond the understanding of children.

Then politics came into our lives. A state of emergency was declared and police trucks roared late at night along the road that led past the university and down the back of the Ridge. I'd once been down there all the way to the end, where the tarmac became patchy and pot-holed and lights on poles lit the gates of the Cato Manor Native Township. I would hear the trucks returning, engines groaning up the hill, and I imagined the prisoners looking through the wire mesh at our house as they were driven past, seeing our lights, and wondered what they felt. Sometimes in the distance there would be sounds like gunshots. In the mornings the road was always empty, with the smell of wet tarmac in the rising heat.

✛

It had rained that morning, making the classrooms dark and forcing us to spend our lunch-break under the dripping trees. Slate-coloured clouds heaped up behind the Ridge and the close air promised more rain on the way. We were back upstairs at our desks when we first heard it; a sort of deep, droning hum that came from far off, filling the room. We looked at Miss Charles, who stared at the buzzing windowpanes with a frown. The doorknob rattled sharply and the teacher leapt up, her face fixed in a rigid smile. She wrenched at the handle, keeping her pale face turned to the class; to comfort us, perhaps, or to prevent an outburst of giggling. The door opened a few inches and the headmaster's hand came through the gap, groping like a blind man's, while he kept up an urgent conversation with someone outside.

'Phone the parents,' we heard him say. 'Tell them to stay at home. The major said it's safest if we remain indoors.'

Then he began to murmur to Miss Charles, who clasped her hands to her chest and looked as if she were going to faint. The boys started to whisper. Some of the girls were drawing shaky breaths and one or two began to cry. Meanwhile, the noise in the distance had risen, become a steady, muted roar. Outside, tyres slid on the wet road. Orders were shouted, boots thumped on the pavement.

'It's the Natives,' declared my friend Rolie, 'they're coming,' and we rushed to the door that led out onto the balcony. Behind us Miss Charles, her legs weighed down by clumps of wailing girls, shouted for us to come back.

We packed the railing, pulling ourselves up to see. The street was full of activity and an assortment of vehicles; ivory-coloured police trucks, traffic-cop motorcycles and a blue bus with wire grilles on the windows were parked randomly across the roadway. The men had been formed into a line below us, naval blue beside policeman grey. They held rifles across their chests and looked from side to side at the men at either shoulder. The motorcycle cops in their boots and jodhpurs clutched pick-handles and fiddled with their pistol-holsters. Grim is the word, I thought, they look grim; but they shifted constantly in their straggling line, swallowing and swallowing. We could feel the plucking hands of the teachers as they tried to get us back indoors, hear their panted orders, but we eluded them, gripping the rails. The line of men began a stiff-legged walk down towards the corner where the street to the school turned up from the main road.

The distant sound had become a collection of individual shouts, a fragmented chanting. We leaned out as far as we could, craning our necks to see what was coming. The cordon of police and soldiers stood with their backs to us, blocking off our street. The sky shifted a notch further towards darkness and the leaves moved sideways in the cool gust before the rain. Suddenly there came the plaintive peep of a car-horn and the ranks divided around a small green Morris that chugged up the road towards the school.

'Hey, Raymond, it's your mom,' shouted someone, 'she's come to get you!'

We could see her anxious face peering up at us through the windscreen as the car wound like a toy between the parked trucks. Raymond flung himself back from the scrum. We heard his shoes clatter down the stairs, his whimpered argument with the woodwork master who guarded the gate below. Then he broke free and hurled his satchel before him through the open window of the moving car, following it in a graceless dive. We watched his thin legs kicking, socks around his ankles, as the little car ground up the hill towards the Ridge.

The rain started, wetting our faces, but none of us took shelter, for a shout had come from the corner. We held our breaths. A shudder seemed to run down the line of men – a collective flinch – as the space beyond them was suddenly filled. One moment we could see the wet roadway between their shoulders and the next it was gone, swallowed up by people, by a mass of dark faces and white shirts, of overalls and umbrellas. I had never seen so many black people at one time; could there be that many in the whole country? The words of their chant came to us clearly. It was in Zulu, strong and deep, familiar sounds that we'd heard around us all our lives. Probably none of us could understand more than a word or two, asking each other: 'What are they saying?'

Rolie nodded sagely. 'You see, it's the women, just like I told you. Whipping them up.'

I listened, but I heard no women's voices, or rather, no voice that stood out clearly enough to say for sure. And no-one really seemed whipped up as they moved past the line of guards, not even glancing at them. Now and then a group would rise up in a sort of bounding dance and then be swallowed again among the crowd, while the mass of people that filled the street continued by, steadily. The warm rain made everything misty, diffused, as though there was glass between us and what was happening. Even the teachers had

HAMPSTEAD PUBLIC LIBRARY

stopped their fretting and stood there with the rest of us, lost in contemplation of this great gathering of strangers in our midst. Perhaps for some of them – for some of us, even – there was a realisation that we might be seeing the future.

When my mother came to pick me up she was glowing with a quiet delight. 'It's happening all over town,' she said. 'I drove right through the crowds. There was no violence, they were perfectly orderly, making way for me. Perhaps there's hope, after all.'

'You were lucky,' I informed her, excited and scared by what I had seen. 'My friend Rolie said they were going to kill us.'

She looked at me, her face suddenly sad.

'Don't listen to those boys,' she said.

The next day we got an armoured car outside our house. It sat square on the patch of grass beneath the streetlamp, its lugged tyres taller than I was, and the gun in the turret pointed up along the road that rose towards the stone gateposts of the university. The vehicle's steel plating had a rough, top-heavy look; too thin, to my well-read eye, to stop anything larger than a two-pounder. The crew were conscripts, I could tell by their shoulder-flashes. Bored, contemptuous, lonely, they sat in their places watching along that strip of tarmac where the heat made flowing lines like water. They may have wondered what it was that they were supposed to be facing, been afraid some of the time, but they were never in doubt of their purpose in being there. They were the front line. They wore pouches of khaki webbing, the same stuff that my dad had brought back from the war, but his old pack that hung behind my bedroom door was sun-bleached and stained with the ghosts of oil-puddles from the streets of Naples and the quays at Port Said. The equipment of these soldiers was stiff and new. I pitied them, that they had seen nothing; would see nothing, for the road stayed obstinately empty.

The following morning they were still there, so I brought them mugs of tea. They let me sit in the turret and swing the machine gun in lazy, inertial arcs. I studied them, their cocksure boredom, and listened to them talk about their homes and the families they were defending. The driver, sitting in the hull of the armoured car, had a transistor radio on the edge of his hatch and I could hear him singing:

'whether it's cloudy
or wet or shine,
if you keep on smiling
it'll turn out fine.
Give a man a Lucky...
– *dang-dang* –
Lucky Strike!'

I was unable to believe that I would ever have a part in a war like this, a war against nothing. No enemy tank, grey and low, would slide its barrel between those gateposts. Only people, walking in their thousands, if they ever came again. At night there was a far-off crackling, the suggestion of a red glow in the sky behind the Ridge, and I thought of the soldiers looking at each other in the dark, listening from within the confines of their cooling armour. Apart from an occasional car returning from a cocktail party in the suburbs, the only things that moved out there were the looping shadows of the flying ants around the white streetlight.

✛

The state of emergency was arresting anyone who was active in politics, and some of my parents' friends started to leave. Rose and Louie decided to give it all up, to go to England or perhaps America. They told us about it over drinks, looking out over the lights reflected in the bay like emigrants dreaming of the Promised Land. On Sunday we went to see them off at the airport. The armoured car had gone during the night, leaving behind cigarette ends and some great rips in the grass, and our Humber rolled down deserted streets past sprinklers that watered the green verges. The black domestic workers, who usually could be found sitting there on their day off in talkative groups, were nowhere to be seen.

The road to the airport skirted the docks and the shunting yards and the quay where the old war-time flying-boat base had been. There were still a couple of derelict Sunderlands, sunk in the shallows. Their wings tilted from the water, shedding white flakes of paint and seagull shit, and I imagined them taxiing out before the dawn in sheets of spray to lift off on patrol, looking for enemy submarines far beyond the place where the brown silt of the river-mouths stained the sea fifty miles out.

The walls of the airport cafeteria were decorated with miniature propellers. We ordered tea that came in thick white cups. I'd asked for a meat pie and was watching the Worcester sauce soak through the crust when the flight was announced. The women embraced, crying. Then Rose hooked her bag over her shoulder and Louie put his arm around her and they walked through the glass doors to where the propeller-wash flattened the grass. We watched the plane bank over the green wall of the Bluff and fly north until it was out of sight.

There was silence for a while on the way back, apart from my mother's sniffing. I touched her shoulder and she gave me a brief smile. She turned to my father.

'Elaine's going too, and the Epsteins. I'm going to miss them terribly.' She squeezed his arm below his rolled-up sleeve. 'We'll be all alone soon. Who's left?'

'Lots of people. I don't know.'

They looked at each other doubtfully.

'Well, let's find out. We'll have a party,' he suggested, and they began to discuss whom they could invite, what the theme should be.

'The Wandering Jew.'

My mother giggled. 'Don't be gauche.'

'Well, look at us; all scattered again, pulling up roots.'

We drove past the shunting yards, jolting over the tracks that ran across the road. They disappeared into the side of a vast, hollow building that had been built to store flour. There was always a light on at the top of one of the towers, behind a dusty window, and I was trying to get my head down far enough to see whether it was there today when I heard my father's sudden intake of breath, like a hiss. Ahead of us the pavement was filled with people pouring out of the gates of the 'Non-Whites Only' football ground. Sports matches weren't allowed on a Sunday, so they must have been at a meeting. After the march I'd witnessed, I couldn't understand why there weren't hundreds of cops around.

'There's not much property here to protect,' said my dad. He pointed at the vacant lots. 'There'll be plain-clothes men among the crowd.' We bumped onto the bridge and he slowed the car to a crawl. Around us the people spilled onto the roadway, closely packed, yet here and there bodies leapt and jostled and ran forward a few steps in unison just like the fluid dance I had seen from the school balcony. The men wore coats and hats, some of the women had black and green cloths tied around their waists. Again I wondered where all these dark faces came from, where they lived: in the hills behind the city, or in the servants' quarters tucked at the bottom of the gardens of the big white homes?

On the bridge there was a violent stir, a surge against the rails, and a man fell into the gutter. At once the crowd broke like a wall, all in the same direction. I thought of air raids, of panicked crowds. The sealed car windows and the rustle of the air-conditioner blocked out all sound. The man in the gutter had pale yellow socks and he lay on his back, one shoe and slender ankle pointing above the curb at the sky. We sat there, vulnerable, ignored, while around us the silent rush continued. I grasped a handful of my father's shirt, feeling the tension in his shoulder muscles. No one looked at my white face pressed against the glass.

✛

The party was a success. Among those that were leaving and the ones who were staying there was the same tense gaiety, a determination to be happy, and some drinks soon had everyone in a fine mood. I met an uncle of mine, a handsome man who had won the Distinguished Flying Cross in a bombing raid on Warsaw and now lived in mysterious circumstances with a woman who was not his wife. He brought his gin and tonic up to my bedroom and correctly identified all the model planes that I had hanging from the ceiling. I liked him, he was someone I could talk to. I showed him my books, a picture of a Wellington bomber like the one he'd flown, and he started to tell me a story about the war but I could see that he was distracted, his ears tuned to the high laugh of his girlfriend Joyce, who held the men enthralled on the veranda below.

'What do you think about them bombing the electricity pylons?' I asked him.

'Oh, that.' He waved his hand dismissively. 'You can hardly call those bombs.' He wore a dark blazer with a crest on the pocket, and I knew he was going to stay. I just wasn't that sure about myself.

'Ever been shot down?' I asked.

'Not yet,' he said, and laughed. 'I have to get back downstairs. Joyce...'

I leaned on the veranda rail, looking down at the guests and the lines of light on the bay. Beyond the cargo-cranes the black bulk of the Bluff cut the sky. On it, I knew, the great coastal defence cannons were trained over the harbour approaches, gathering dew. They were useless now, for the onslaught would come from their backs, from the dark valleys behind the Ridge. The anti-aircraft guns were there too, wasted, forever without enemy bombers to make them flash and recoil on their mountings. From the party below came a great gust of warmth and laughter. I watched the shadows of my war-planes turn slowly against the ceiling.

✪

It was by no means clear where this military interest came from. I was not descended out of warrior stock. My ancestors were traders and scholars from Eastern Europe, Lithuania and Russia, feeble as fighters even in self-defence against the Cossacks who raged through their villages in drunken pogroms. After the assassination of the Tsar by revolutionaries in 1881 these attacks became more systematic and deadly, and it seemed wisest to seek a future elsewhere. My grandparents separately had ended up in South Africa, where they'd met and married. When we had dinner at their house I'd sit in the lounge on the pale green carpet – the same colour as the rare hydrangeas my grandmother cultivated – and explore their bookshelves. Many of the books I couldn't understand. Some were in Russian or Yiddish or German, and there were English ones with puzzling titles like *The Intelligent Man's Guide to Jew-Baiting*. My grandfather was a big man with iron-grey hair and pink hearing aids that were connected by plaited wires to a box in his shirt-pocket. Conversation with him was difficult, and it was only many years later that I was able to put together the story of his youth.

Aged ten, he'd been sent to America; put on a ship in Riga bound for New York with a pouch around his neck containing money and the address of an uncle in Grand Rapids, Michigan. Some years there and in Detroit taught him English and something about business, while leaving him partly deaf from an attack of meningitis. At sixteen, alone and self-reliant, he sailed for South Africa to seek his fortune, arriving towards the end of the Anglo-Boer War. Boer horseback *kommandos* still staged guerrilla raids in the countryside, but Johannesburg had fallen to the British and he set up there as a coal-merchant, heaving the sacks on his broadening shoulders.

In 1905 he'd moved to the British colony of Natal, first to Durban and then to the small farming community of Mooi River, where he took the job of managing the Argyle Hotel. Now nineteen years old, my grandfather would ride each week to Pietermaritzburg to collect the mail, a day's journey in either direction, with a rifle across his saddle to protect himself and his horse from lions. The hotel bar had a long mirror that was smashed periodically by the revolver-shots of drunken farmers. Each time, a replacement had to be brought by ox-wagon from Durban. It took weeks to arrive and might be broken again as soon as it was installed; the farmers were in a celebratory mood as they enlarged their meat and dairy holdings inland and planted sugar along the coast. But among the Zulus, whose land was being taken, there was growing anger.

Then a poll-tax was imposed – payable in pounds sterling – aimed at forcing the Zulus to work on the white man's farms or down the mines. By the start of 1906 it was clear that open rebellion threatened. The colonial authorities seemed set on confrontation, handing out whippings and imprisonment to those who did not pay. Bambata, a minor chief, remembered the great Zulu nation of King Cetshwayo before it had been smashed by the British army twenty-seven years before. He declared that his clan would pay no tax and ambushed the column of Natal Mounted Police sent to his kraal to arrest him, killing four troopers. A number of other tribal chiefs joined Bambata's cause. Settlers in outlying areas abandoned their properties and fled to the towns. All able-bodied white men were called upon to join the colonial militia, to defend Pietermaritzburg and Durban from the Zulu hordes. My grandfather rode in from Mooi River and volunteered for a soldier.

It was fortunate, from a moral point of view, that his deafness made him unsuitable for service. Bambata's uprising was a tragedy. The authorities declared martial law and mobilised an overwhelming force of cavalry, infantry regiments, machine-gun batteries and field artillery. Bambata and his followers were hunted down and surrounded in the Nkandhla Forest, where they had retreated to the sacred valley that was the burial place of the Zulu kings. Artillery, quick-firing cannon and Maxim guns rained down fire from the heights. Riflemen blazed away with dum-dum bullets. Hundreds of rebels fell around Cetshwayo's grave, an unknown number more dying of their wounds in the forest, while the government forces suffered only a handful of casualties. Bambata's body was found among the slain and his head cut off, to be displayed as proof that the rebellion was dead. It had cost the lives of some thirty whites and over three thousand blacks. A silver Bambata Rebellion campaign medal was struck for the victors. Dinizulu, Cetshwayo's son and heir to what remained of his dismantled kingdom, was imprisoned – though he'd dissociated himself from the uprising – in order to crush the final vestiges of Zulu nationhood. And, no matter in so iniquitous a cause, my grandfather had offered to serve.

2

Desert Fever

At the end of our first week on the kibbutz we were issued with rifles. They were heavy and long, almost as long as we were, and a lot older: Mausers, manufactured in the early forties in Nazi-occupied Czechoslovakia, stamped with the eagle and swastika of the German Wehrmacht and then over-stamped with the Hebrew initials of the Tsvah Haganah L'Yisrael, the Israeli Defence Force. We each drew one of these scarred old veterans from the armoury, plus a flat tin cleaning-kit with an oil bottle that leaked a creosote-scented sludge, and sat in rows on the ground to be shown the techniques of field-care: tugging an oil-soaked patch of cloth down the barrel with the pull-through cord and stripping the mechanism of the rifle-bolt to wipe the dust from its greased components.

I was fourteen years old and these manoeuvres were for real. The year before, in 1967, Israel had vanquished its Arab neighbours with lightning efficiency in the Six-Day War. Newsreels showed columns of black smoke standing above the desert and Egyptian MiGs blitzed on their runways in pre-emptive air strikes that had disassembled them into component parts, like model aeroplane kits. Internationally, Israel's standing was high; even in South Africa. The bruisers from the Afrikaner high-school against whom we played football still hacked viciously at our shins, but they had dropped their hisses of 'Jewboy' in acknowledgement of our kinship with Moshe Dayan, the conquering general with the black eye-patch. The Hebrew song 'Jerusalem the Golden' played again and again on Springbok Radio. Its haunting threnody formed the soundtrack of patriotic evenings at the Durban Jewish Club, where the community held collections for war bonds and watched film of young paratroopers, helmets clutched against their chests, weeping at the Wailing Wall.

A group of us from Durban were to have the privilege (subsidised by proud parents) of making the *aliyah,* the pilgrimage to Israel, in her time of triumph. We would be doing pioneer work – I was to spend four months on a kibbutz in the Negev Desert – and my mother took me round the shops to equip me. At Mahomadies, the town's big Indian-owned outfitters, I got twill shirts and heavy canvas trousers that would keep their rigidity even after being beaten on stones. Despite the courteous assistance of the son-in-law who served us, I knew that it would be insensitive to mention the reason for these purchases; in the prelude to the Six-Day War, as hostilities loomed, Durban's Muslim population had donated blood that was flown to Arab capitals and used subsequently to treat the many wounded. Their businesses were since being boy-cotted by some of the town's Jews, but these Muslim families were my father's patients and he made no such distinction.

Reticence was unnecessary at Woolfson's clothing emporium, which supplied me with lace-up work boots and a heavy leather jacket. I showed it to my grandfather for his imprimatur. After the Bambata Rebellion he had continued running the hotel until he'd accumulated a sufficient stake to start a business, eventually pros-pering in Durban as a dealer in hides and leather which he exported to Italy. Peering through his thick spectacles, the old man stroked the fleece lining with his thumb.

'Merino, first quality,' he said. 'A good buy.'

I examined it too and saw that the pile was backed with cloth.

'It's synthetic,' I informed him.

He shook his head, betrayed by his fingers that had once graded pelts so infallibly. I wondered at the urge for truth that had gripped me. The passport issued to me for the journey showed a boy I didn't really recognise, in heavy black-framed spectacles, who stared from the photograph with a somewhat chubby intensity.

Our party from Durban, along with kids from Cape Town, Port Elizabeth and East London, flew to Johannesburg, where the larg-est contingent came from. We met for the first time at the airport on the evening of our departure. Parents sobbed and clutched at their departing teenagers while younger siblings, over-excited by the late hour, dashed about underfoot. Despite my loneliness I was relieved that I had got my farewells behind me in Durban. Soon after take-off I fell asleep, woken intermittently by high-spirited yells and excruciating sing-songs. We landed at dawn at Israel's Lod International Airport, and our group of some forty boys and girls was herded onto the bus that would take us to the kibbutz. The road ran through green hills and then swung south, and I watched from a window seat as the landscape gradually transformed itself into a place of utter foreignness.

This was my first time truly away from home, and I knew nothing. I'd never experienced hunger or significant illness, or any degree of real discomfort. I was accustomed to Durban's humidity, its air saturated with the hothouse smells of greenery and tropical sea. The desert was a shock; a plain of chalk that glared in the harsh light. The sky burned pink like a gas flame. After a couple of hours the bus swung off the main road and onto a track that led to the kibbutz. Apart from a vivid patch of irrigated lawn at the community centre and the dusty leaves of the orange groves, every colour lay in the spectrum of beige. We were unloaded before a concrete structure in a weighty neo-bunker style that I later discovered was the vernacular for all Israeli public buildings from the national Parliament downwards. The settlement's heart comprised two residential streets and a park of landscaped mounds and eucalyptus saplings around a children's play area, deserted in the midday heat. From the eating hall came a clatter of steel.

Our quarters were a row of just-constructed concrete houses on the settlement's edge; a stack of prefab panels around a clotted cement mixer marked the next one to be built. Beyond it, two lines of kerbstones ran out into the dust towards where the wire of the perimeter fence glinted in the sun. Eight or ten of us were assigned to each house – one was for the girls – and we rushed in to claim our beds. An enervating heat permeated the interiors, radiating down through the flat roofs. I ended up sharing a room with two other boys from Durban: stocky Ivan the Intelligent, whose father was a psychiatrist, and Polmeier, a gentle lad who already wore the hangdog face of homesickness. The others in our house came from Cape Town. The front room was claimed by Ishie: small, sharp-featured, with a cynic's wit, at fourteen already the man he would be for the rest of his life. He shared with disdainful Zimmy – a Seapoint sophisticate who wore tasselled loafers instead of workboots – and wiry Morris, who could have been Ishie's twin, a complainer and comic, irreverent and deeply conservative. Sam, known as Shmully, occupied the other room with Bobo and Wayne: one loud, one quiet, one plump and devout.

Those in the house next door were all from Johannesburg. Their leader was Tubmann, a well-built chap with dark hair and the beginnings of chin-stubble, who looked after – with brusque condescension – the witless Norm, as big as he was but running to fat. Both wore yarmulkes on their heads and were recent converts to the religious youth movement called B'nai Akivah. Two believers named Aaron were among the rest of the household of Tubmann's sidekicks, whom he bullied and patronised in equal measure. That night we joined the rest of the kibbutz community for our inaugural meal, the first – and, as it would turn out, the best – of our planned four-month stay. Before each place at the long tables stood paired plastic beakers. One contained black coffee, the other – in acknowledgement of the fact that it was Friday night – sweet Sabbath wine. I slugged at the two alternately while the welcome speeches droned. Ishie and Ivan topped up my cups and I found myself, for the first time in my young life, experiencing a tipsy alertness that was hugely enjoyable. My euphoria was disturbed by Tubmann, who threatened to bash me for my 'lack of respect'. I resolved to avoid him as much as possible.

✛

The kibbutz was called Sde Boqer ('The Fields of Morning', or perhaps 'of the Cowboys'), and had a special symbolic significance in a country dense with symbols. It had been established in 1952 as a pioneer outpost on the edge of the desolate lands called the Wilderness of Zin, once the southern border of the biblical kingdom of Judea. The kibbutz's legendary resident was David Ben-Gurion, founder of the State of Israel in 1948 and its first prime minister, whose life-story was that of Zionism itself. Born the same year as my grandfather, in a *shtetl* across the border in Poland, he'd arrived in Palestine in 1906 to work as a farmhand and begun organising Jewish workers into the socialist Federation of Jewish Labour. Initially the Zionist Left claimed that there was no conflict between the interests of Jewish workers and those of Palestinian Arabs, whose shared struggle was against their class enemy, the Ottoman landowners. But Ben-Gurion watched Arab resistance grow as the twenties and thirties brought ever more Jews to Palestine, and he split the socialist Labour movement away from the communists – with their utopian dreams of a binational Jewish-Arab state – and began building a defence organisation, the Haganah, to protect settler lands.

He also had to deal with the hard-right Zionist Revisionists, established in 1925 by a militant Jewish nationalist named Ze'ev Jabotinsky. In Palestine the Revisionists provided military training and formed an underground army, the Irgun: 'Zionism is a colonisation adventure,' explained Jabotinsky, 'and therefore it stands or falls on the question of armed force.' The Revisionist underground was ruthless, if not always logical. In 1933 it assassinated as a 'collaborator' the head of the Labour movement, who had visited officials in Nazi Germany to negotiate the migration of Jews to Palestine. The Irgun also targeted Palestine's British administration for trying to limit Jewish settlement, and once the Second World War began, Revisionists made contact with both Mussolini and the Nazi Foreign Office through the Vichy French government in Syria, offering to fight on the Axis side in exchange for the guarantee of a post-war Jewish State. In 1944 the Irgun's commander Menachem Begin called for all Jews in Palestine to rise up against the British, while Revisionist underground members assassinated Lord Moyne, the British minister-resident in Cairo.

The result was disastrous to Jewish unity. Winston Churchill, who had long been sympathetic to Zionism, now condemned it for producing 'a new set of gangsters worthy of Nazi Germany' and the Jewish authorities in Palestine handed over the names of some seven hundred Irgun members to the British, who arrested them. But Revisionist attacks continued. In 1946 they blew up the King David Hotel in Jerusalem, killing ninety – Jews, Arabs and British – and during Israel's 1948 War of Independence they assassinated the UN negotiator Count Bernadotte, who was trying to arrange a ceasefire agreement that would halt the fighting. Denouncing Revisionist forces as terrorists, Prime Minister Ben-Gurion ordered them disbanded, whereupon Irgun leader Menachem Begin and other Revisionists formed a hard-right opposition party in the Israeli parliament.

Its continuing attacks on Ben-Gurion were among the reasons for his decision in 1953 to resign as prime minister and move to Sde Boqer, exhausted by what he described as the 'morbid fragmentation' of Israeli politics. In and out of government as minister of defence and again as prime minister, he led his country through the 1956 Suez War and gave up the premiership for the last time in 1963 to retire to Sde Boker. Shortly after our arrival at the kibbutz we were taken to see him where he sat on his veranda: now eighty-two, a portly man with hair as white as his shirt, who lectured us in richly accented English about the need for national watchfulness as we sat below on his bungalow lawn.

Sde Boqer was a 'youth' kibbutz that provided overseas visitors with an immersion in the Hebrew language and some experience of communal living. Our group of South Africans joined other youngsters already in residence – Americans, Canadians, a few English – who had been there long enough to absorb the unassailable self-confidence and patriotism of native Israelis. Over the next days we began to learn the features of this egalitarian community: the use of first names to address our seniors, the gatherings for *mitz* – synthetic orange juice – a couple of times a day, duty permitting, and the evening get-togethers called *kumsitz;* part discussion group, part sing-along. Most of the kids I was with knew all the words to the pioneer songs, having been members of the Jewish youth organisation *Habonim* – 'the Builders' – back in South Africa. I'd been a Boy Scout instead, and couldn't contribute.

At the *kumsitz* we met Barak, a muscular sixty-five-year-old with a moustache yellowed from the smoke of the Russian cigarette whose cardboard mouthpiece was clamped always between his teeth. He had survived the Nazi death camp at Sobibor – a fading number was tattooed on his forearm – to reach Israel in 1947 on one of the illegal refugee ships that penetrated the Royal Navy's blockade. Spirited off the beach before British patrols could catch them, the new arrivals were assigned to remote kibbutzes. Barak been sent to the Huleh Valley north of Lake Galilee to work chest-deep in water, 'draining ze svamps,' until he was called up to fight.

We sat in the dark around the coal of Barak's cigarette while he taught us the words of the plaintive Arabic song called 'Bab el Wadh' – 'The Gate of the Valley' – the name of the narrow defile between the hills that guarded the road to Jerusalem. Through the 1948 Israeli War of Independence the song had been sung by both sides, contesting the valley in repeated, bitter fighting. Barak's Haganah unit had been directed to capture its key position, the Jordanian-held ex-British police fort at Latrun. The attackers ran up the road carrying a large kitchen table, which they'd placed against the outer wall of the fort as an improvised firing step, pouring gunfire and grenades into the compound until heavy losses had forced their withdrawal. Barak had been wounded in that engagement and seen comrades fall, but twenty years on, his true enmity was reserved for Revisionist 'terrorists'. With the point of his cigarette he punctured the myth of the final moments of Josef Trumpeldor, the man whose death had been the inspiration for Jabotinsky's Zionist Revisionist movement. Trumpeldor had come to Palestine after Russian army service in the 1904 Russo-Japanese War, served alongside Jabotinsky during World War One in a British army Jewish volunteer unit called the Zion Mule Corps and been killed in 1920 defending his kibbutz from an Arab attack.

'Zey say Trumpeldor's last vords vos, "it is good to die for vun's country",' growled Barak around the cardboard tube of his smoke, 'but vot he really said vos, "fuck, it hurts".'

Several of the boys bridled. 'That's bullshit,' declared Tubmann, and beside me the Aarons muttered angrily.

Barak examined them over his great moustache. 'So.' he nodded. 'Terrorists, baby terrorists.' It seemed that the schism was alive yet.

✪

Sde Boqer housed the National Desert School, established to study the ecology and archaeology of the Negev. There was a department of anthropology that recorded the lives of the Bedouin nomads to whom this region had once been home. During the War of Independence many had fled, their return prevented by the minefields and barbed wire that grew along the borders with Egypt to the west and Jordan in the east. By the end of the war Israel controlled the entire Negev down to the Red Sea, and kept the triangle of desert under military administration until 1965 – some years after it had ceased in other areas of Israel – in order to complete the removal of the remaining twenty-six thousand Negev Bedouin from lands required for Jewish settlement. Forced into 'compulsory townships' around Beersheba, their nomadic past remained commemorated in the form of a gloomy diorama in the Desert School museum, where plaster figures in burnouses crouched under a black goat's-wool tent around a fire-effect of twigs piled on an orange light-bulb.

David, a young archaeologist from the school, took a group of us into the desert. Two and a half thousand years before, this harsh land had been cultivated by the Nabataeans, whose capital had been at Petra across the Jordanian border, and he was studying the techniques they'd used to save the waters of the periodic flash floods that tore down the dry wadis. Striding through the sand in scuffed paratroop boots, his black curls jammed under an old slouch-hat, David pointed out ancient terraces and the entrances to underground cisterns hewn in the sandstone. Few other signs remained of that once-flourishing civilisation, apart from the ancient mound of Tel Yeruham some miles to the north of the kibbutz. Here a dig was in progress, exposing Nabataean ruins among strata of settlement going back into pre-history. I volunteered for spade-work in the trenches, shifting mounds of dirt, in the hope of being excused Hebrew lessons. It didn't work.

The classrooms were baking prefabs whose wall-panels clattered in the desert wind. Flies droned around our heads and settled on the textbooks, where, to stay awake, I killed them methodically, lining up their corpses along the desk edge. I had great difficulty reading Hebrew, especially the demotic form written without vowels, and would spend the lesson laboriously pencilling phonetic renderings above each word in anticipation that I might be asked to read aloud. I looked forward to travelling around the country, when I would be able to try speaking the language rather than speculating on its pronunciation. In the meantime I hoped that the communal labour we had been told was part of our kibbutz sojourn would provide some respite from the classroom, but it turned out that enough time could be made in each day both to water orange trees and to learn Hebrew, as well as performing the other duties that life on the settlement demanded of us.

☉

The kibbutz stood on the edge of a spectacular gorge of pink and ochre sandstone. A few miles along it a waterfall plunged into a pool, overlooked by cells cut into the rocks by hermit monks a thousand years before. Beyond, the wilderness stretched eastwards to where it dropped into the Wadi Arabah – that part of the Great Rift Valley running south from the Dead Sea – that formed the border with Jordan. There was a track up the escarpment called Ma'alei Akhrabim, the 'Ascent of the Scorpion,' an historic trading road overlooked by the ruins of ancient fortifications. More recently it had been used as an infiltration route by Palestinian gunmen attacking targets inside Israel – in revenge for Israeli army raids into Jordan that had been retaliation for previous attacks – in a cycle of blood feud that was interrupted only by periodic escalations into full-scale war.

In this atmosphere of perpetual tension, isolated kibbutzes like Sde Boqer were responsible for their own defence. All of us, girls as well as boys, were taught how to handle our rifles. Belly-down on canvas groundsheets, we practised to the instructor's orders. *One:* click-clatter of the bolt pulled open; *two:* rattle as a clip of five (deactivated) bullets were stuck into the receiver; *three:* squeak of the magazine-spring, compressed by the cartridges thumbed down into the magazine; *four:* bolt slammed closed, flicking away the empty clip and carrying the first round into the breach. 'Rifle loaded and locked,' we shouted in ragged Hebrew harmony. Unloading, we kept the weapon to our shoulders as though firing and worked the bolt as fast as we could, spinning away the ejected cartridges until the bolt stuck open to reveal the empty breach. 'Rifle open and clean,' we yelled.

The ballet over, we would go wandering about the training area to reclaim our cartridges, wipe off the sand and stick them back in their clips before repeating the drill. We were also required to throw practice grenades, though I found that even my wildest fling – almost dislocating my elbow – could not propel the heavy lumps of lead far enough to avoid their theoretical kill zone. We did press-ups and pull-ups, chanting our counts higher and higher until they became grunts of pain. The instructors made us run the obstacle course again and again, cutting down our time, and though I never again found a use for the wide-stepped dance along a plain of motorcar tyres, or arm-swinging from rung to rung beneath a horizontal ladder, I've been saved subsequently by the trick we were taught to spring ourselves over the high wall.

For shooting instruction we were taken to a rifle range in the desert beyond the settlement. We used Mausers rebarrelled to .22 and tried to hit the speck of a target that swam in the heat-haze. Beside us the officers and instructors would be firing automatic weapons in ripping bursts that set our pulses racing and unsettled our aim. The sights on the rifles were pretty bashed about and the results already haphazard enough, though I did once win a bronze marksman's badge for grouping five shots in the bit of tape that secured one corner of the target card.

Each night a half-dozen of us would be detailed to go out on patrol. After the evening meal we'd report to the armoury to draw a rifle and equipment belt carrying two water-bottles, which we filled from the tank. The officer who would lead the night patrol – during the day he might be a tractor driver or kibbutz electrician or an academic at the Desert School – checked that we were wearing dark clothes and suitable boots and that our equipment didn't glint or rattle. Then we filed through a gate in the perimeter fence and out into the desert.

The patrols were intended to apply the tactics of the original Special Night Squads, established by the Haganah as a means of kibbutz defence in the 1930s. These small units, trained to move and communicate in the dark, would circle away from their settlements and set up ambushes along likely approach routes used by raiders, in order to attack the attackers. To this end we needed to learn basic star navigation and have instilled in us some concept of march discipline. We had to move in silence, speaking only to pass along the column whispered direction-changes or warnings of obstacles; it took Ivan the Intelligent a while to learn not to simply say, 'I know,' when – apparently self-evident – orders reached him for transmission onwards. At rest halts we'd drink in turn from one water-bottle until it had been emptied, so that no sloshing sound would give away our presence as we walked.

Although it was not intended that we should be put at risk, these patrols also had the security function of checking for nocturnal activity in the surrounding desert, and the squad leader carried a submachine gun and a pack containing ammunition for our Mausers. The marches covered many miles. Lights were forbidden; instead we were taught to use every bit of natural illumination. Objects could be defined by dropping flat to silhouette them against the starlit sky. In the valleys were hummocks of leafless scrub that tripped us up; they could be avoided by watching for the snail-shells that glowed like phosphorescence amidst their roots. We climbed the ridges with care, trying to avoid the flints underfoot sparking in the dry air. At each crest we would lie amidst the rocks to study the next wadi for movement. With all the fervour of youth I loved these night patrols; the excitement of new skills, the mouth-drying apprehension at a sudden noise.

There were other nights when we stood guard instead, for four-hour shifts out on the kibbutz perimeter fence. This was both duller and more frightening than patrolling, for shadows appeared to move if you stared too long and the tins hung on the wire would sometimes stir without a breath of wind, causing the stones inside them to clunk and rattle. Many of our contingent avoided this duty by sleeping on the roofs of their houses, where they would not be found and roused by the guard officer. Sustained by a solitary delight, I did my stints.

From a security and economic viewpoint the country remained on a war footing. Quality produce was being exported to pay off war loans. Whatever was in glut or of a standard too poor for the domestic market was trucked to the kibbutzes, and the food was consequently dire. Chicken happened on Friday nights. At midweek, to keep up our protein levels, we received 'the escalope', a sheet of unspecified animal cased in gritty breadcrumbs. For a period we subsisted on pre-sliced white bread and avocado pears for two meals a day; a great bin of them stood in the eating hall, through which we picked to try to find those that were not black and liquefied. We ate avocado with sugar and lemon juice, with black pepper and lemon juice, with salt and lemon juice. Despite our heat-vitiated appetites we were always hungry. When the last of the avocados, too advanced in decay to be eaten, were pitched to the pigs, processed cheese squares took their place. These were welded onto bread by a great conveyor-belt toaster capable of preparing a hundred slices a minute, that emerged – crusts smoking, cheese billowing in milky blisters – on steel trays. It was advisable not to take a portion on which a blister had not collapsed, for some bumps concealed the bodies of fleshy cockroaches.

Kids started to get sick. In our house, Wayne came down with gastro-enteritis. The city plumpness melted away and his weight plummeted, turning him to a haggard ghost who trailed a sour, fishy smell that I learned later at medical school was diagnostic of giardiasis. People retreated from Wayne, holding their noses. Knowing that I ought to feel compassion, I avoided him too, for his misery and the pathetic inclination of his head were unbearable to see. He was taken eventually to the sick-bay, where Ivan prevailed upon a group of us to visit him. We arrived as the medic was sticking an intravenous infusion in his arm with a needle of impressive calibre. He used another to inject the contents of an ampoule of Vitamin B into Wayne's buttock. I felt decidedly queasy. The others looked pale, but bravely identified me to the kibbutz nurse as the son of a doctor.

'Good,' she said, 'you stay and keep count.' She showed me how to adjust the rate of the infusion with a little wheel that controlled the number of drops. I watched the bubbles dancing in the transparent drip-chamber, wishing that I could be elsewhere. I was repelled by Wayne's whimpering and wondered how doctors managed to maintain sympathy for the suffering. If this was what practicing medicine involved, I was not the sort to volunteer.

✚

My father had been different. After graduating from medical school at the end of 1940 he'd elected to join the South African Army Medical Corps, then asked to be sent on active service 'up north' (all South Africans who served outside the borders of their country during the war did so as volunteers) and been despatched in a troopship to join a forward field hospital. He had eventually been demobilised in England in 1945, with the rank of captain and extensive experience in orthopaedic surgery, which he decided would be his specialist field. Finding a post in an English hospital, he studied for and obtained the Fellowship examination of the Royal College of Surgeons. His friends included a group of Jewish ex-servicemen, and as 1947 ended they were increasingly preoccupied by events in Palestine, where the British administration was preparing its withdrawal.

A November UN vote to partition the country had been denounced as theft of their land by Palestinian Arabs, who attacked Jewish targets. In March 1948 the Haganah responded with an offensive to secure all the areas allocated as Jewish territory under the UN plan, as well as to reinforce Jewish settlements outside these areas and create corridors connecting them as a basis for future Jewish sovereignty. Generalised fighting began, with the British under fire from both sides. Arab villages overlooked the Jerusalem road where it entered the Judaean hills at Bab el Wadh, and Palestinian riflemen, helped by Jordanian artillery, interrupted the passage of Jewish traffic. Jewish West Jerusalem, the Jewish Quarter of the Old City in East Jerusalem and the Hadassah Hospital on Mount Scopus became separate, besieged enclaves. On 22 March the road was cut completely and two weeks passed before a convoy of trucks managed to break through to Jerusalem, with heavy losses. Vicious fighting followed as Haganah forces tried to capture the hills above the road by frontal assault. April 1948 became notorious for two atrocities. Revisionist units attacked the Arab village of Deir Yassin close to Jerusalem's western edge and massacred 245 inhabitants, most of them women and children. In retaliation a convoy of armoured buses was ambushed on its way to the Hadassah Hospital and 75 Jewish doctors, nurses and patients were killed.

Israeli statehood was declared on 14 May 1948 as the last British units left Palestine. At once a struggle began for control of the bases and police posts they had vacated. The armies of Lebanon, Syria, Iraq, Jordan and Egypt advanced into Palestine, refusing to recognise the borders of the new state. Fighting intensified along the Jerusalem road, centred around the ex-British police fort at Latrun, now held by troops of the Jordanian Legion. Jewish immigrants arriving off the ships – concentration camp survivors from Displaced Persons centres in Europe, others just released from British internment camps in Cyprus – were rushed to the Latrun sector and thrown into a disastrous attack. A second attack a few days later – the one in which Barak, our veteran at Sde Boqer, had been wounded – failed too. The Jewish Quarter of the Old City fell. Conditions inside Jewish West Jerusalem were desperate. Improvised armoured vehicles – rough affairs made from sheet-steel, welded around the chassis of a car or truck – attempted to break through the siege lines. Only a few from each convoy managed to reach the city with their vital supplies of food, ammunition and manpower. With Syrian forces attacking in the north and Egyptian armour advancing on Tel Aviv, a call went out to Jewish ex-soldiers internationally to come and help.

Many were no doubt horrified at the idea of going back to war. Some would have settled into peacetime careers, but saw it as their duty. And there were a few who had never readjusted to peace and leapt at the chance to rediscover the camaraderie of service. I can't be sure into which of these categories my father fitted, but when the phone rang one night in early June and he was asked to report to an address the next morning in central London, he went. Four days later he was at an airfield outside the city with a group of other volunteers. The passport in his pocket carried visa number twelve issued by the new Israeli embassy in London, allowing him permission to enter their recently founded country.

He also carried a wedge of other papers. The Haganah had formed the nucleus of an armoured corps by buying three latest-model Centurion tanks from an amenable sergeant at a Haifa army depot during the confusion of the British withdrawal, and they needed the technical blueprints – ordnance, hydraulic, mechanical and electrical – to keep these complex machines running. Someone in England had managed to obtain a set of the bulky documents, which were now being transported to Israel. The volunteers expected the authorities to try to block their journey and were fearful of being searched; some were on the Reserve List of officers in the British armed forces and could be charged with treason under military law. The charts and manuals were divided between the two tallest men, wrapped around their legs beneath their trousers and stuffed inside their shirts. Thus it was that my dad walked, stiff-legged behind a screen of his comrades, past surly UK customs men and up the steps into the aircraft – an ex-military DC3 transport repainted in the livery of 'Pan African Airlines' – that would be carrying them 'on holiday' to the South of France.

The aircraft landed in Paris and then Marseilles, where they slept. The following day they flew to Rome, touching down at an airfield north of the city. A second aircraft arrived carrying volunteers, and my father recognised the pilot as a fellow South African he'd known while stationed as a medical officer at Air Transport Command, who had gone on to fly bombers in the RAF. The pilot offered him a place in the cockpit. Just before dusk the planes took off steeply and were soon flying high above the nightbound Apennines. The Russian blockade around Berlin had been in place for two months, the city surviving on a British and American airlift. Europe was divided into armed camps with both sides on high alert. Searchlights probed the sky. To avoid being detected by air patrols the pilot had to fly at maximum height and soon the men in the body of the plane were blacking out from lack of oxygen. They flew onward over Yugoslavia and Greece – my dad sharing the co-pilot's oxygen mask – with their unconscious cargo.

While they'd been en route to Israel a temporary truce had come in to effect, organised by the United Nations mediator Count Folke Bernadotte. Its terms specified that neither side was to use the four-week ceasefire to bring in men or military equipment. This period saw the arrival of many of the five thousand Mahal (international volunteers) who would come to the country to serve in Israel's

Haganah Defence Force during the War of Independence, plus large quantities of arms – from fighter planes to Mauser rifles – supplied by Czechoslovakia. The arrival of my father's group was camouflaged through a simple ruse; as the planes touched down at an airfield near Haifa a siren began to shriek and anti-aircraft guns opened up along the perimeter. They continued firing skyward while the passengers ran to cover and the aircraft turned around. As soon as they were airborne the gunfire stopped and the new arrivals were welcomed, while Israel made a formal protest to the UN that the ceasefire had been threatened by an attempted Egyptian air-raid.

The truce was precarious. The vehicle in which my father travelled from Haifa to Tel Aviv came under fire, and the only safe way into Jerusalem remained by armoured car. Once there, he was taken to view the Old City's Damascus Gate from a Haganah forward observation post reached through the monastery of Notre Dame, its floors spread with carpets to deaden footsteps; any sound attracted a hail of grenades from the Jordanian Legionnaires over the wall. Jewish deaths during the truce arose too from factional fighting when the *Altalena*, a ship loaded with Irgun arms and volunteers, reached the coast of Israel. Ben-Gurion ordered that the weapons and personnel be disembarked to be incorporated into the Israeli army. On board was the Irgun commander Begin, who refused. Ben-Gurion ordered Haganah forces to seize the vessel. Irgunists on board opened fire on the soldiers ashore, who shot back, setting the ship alight and killing some fighters as they swam to safety.

Returning from Jerusalem, my father reported to the ex-British army hospital in Haifa, now designated Israel's Military Hospital Number Ten. It was full of wounded and almost without equipment, for on their departure the British had dumped into the harbour all that they could not carry away. Standards of care were abysmal, with patients dying from poor surgical technique and sepsis. Compound leg fractures – penetrating wounds that exposed the broken bone to infection – were being treated routinely by amputation. No-one appeared to have knowledge of the Tobruk splint that had saved so many legs in North Africa and other theatres of operations in the Second World War. A welder was found and my dad showed him how to construct the splints, allowing the wounds to be cared for while the underlying fractures healed with traction; a saddler made the leather padding that prevented splint pressure. At night, if my father wasn't operating, the three of them would raid the building sites of Haifa to steal iron reinforcing rods from which these simple, limb-saving devices could be made. With other doctors he set up a blood cross-matching laboratory and transfusion service for the treatment of casualties suffering major blood-loss. Operating facilities improved when a diver brought to the hospital handfuls of surgical instruments that he'd found at the bottom of Haifa Harbour.

The truce ended on 8 July and fresh casualties streamed into Military Hospital Number Ten as fighting resumed on all fronts. Settlements to the south of Tel Aviv held out against renewed Egyptian attacks. There were Israeli successes in the northern sector, where the Haganah eventually took Nazareth amidst reports of soldiers looting buildings they had captured instead of seeing to their defence, so that they were temporarily beaten back by Arab counter-attacks. Fortunes on the central front were mixed. The Arab Legion forces holding Lydda Airport – later to be Lod International, where I would land two decades later – were forced to retreat by the Centurion tanks for which the operating manuals had been brought from England, but two more failed attacks on Latrun brought heavy Israeli casualties. The Mahal doctors worked ceaselessly; one South African surgeon entered the operating room on 18 July and emerged thirty-six hours later, having operated on twenty-eight wounded in succession.

By then the UN mediator had managed to negotiate a second ceasefire, but Revisionist units in Jerusalem rejected the truce and kept fighting. They also assassinated Count Bernadotte and a French UN officer, credited during the war with saving Jews from Nazi deportation. The bodies were brought to the Haifa military hospital, where my father was one of the officers detailed to witness the autopsies. Finding that epaulettes and buttons had been cut off the dead men's uniforms by a mortuary assistant to sell as souvenirs, he ordered that they be restored. Amidst a mood of national disgust Ben-Gurion instructed the Revisionist units to be dissolved and their forces merged with the Haganah, though the assassins would never be brought to justice.

New weapons arrived, including armour and heavy bombers, and in mid-October the re-equipped Israeli forces broke the ceasefire and pressed forward to seize their territorial objectives. Driving the Egyptians out of Beersheba in Operation Ten Plagues, they advanced southwards into the Negev, leaving an enemy brigade surrounded at Faluja which, with young Major Gamal Abdul Nasser among its commanders, fell only after a bitter two-month siege. On the northern front Mahal volunteers under a Canadian colonel defeated the Syrian army and Arab irregulars to take the region of the Upper Galilee. Casualties, brought straight to Haifa, received swift, effective treatment. The war ended in March 1949 with the Israelis occupying the Negev down to the Gulf of Aqaba, securing an outlet to the Red Sea. Desperate attacks had widened the Jerusalem Corridor but the Old City remained in Jordanian hands, as did the strategic Latrun fort.

Throughout the conflict the resourceful doctors at Military Hospital Number Ten had devised new methods of treatment to improve the survival of the wounded and the outcome of their injuries. My father stayed on after the armistice was signed, serving a year and a half in Israel as an army surgeon. He was always busy; there was much reconstructive surgery to be done. One day he met a vivacious young woman doctor who had arrived from South Africa with a load of medical supplies.

'He was tall, suntanned, lean as a wolf,' she later recalled. 'He had a car, and the first outing he took me on was a smuggling expedition: buying suitcase-loads of eggs from the Druze villages on the slopes of Mt Carmel and dodging the military police checkpoints to bring them back to the hospital, so the patients would have some protein in their diets for their wounds to heal.'

Three years later, back in Durban, they were married.

✪

Now, in 1968, twenty years after my dad had travelled to Jerusalem during the War of Independence's first, uncertain ceasefire, I was following his journey, passing the rusted shells of armoured cars left as monuments beside the road that they had fought to keep open. In West Jerusalem I stayed with relatives in their modern apartment and wandered the Old City's alleyways of golden stone. Arab homes were being bulldozed in the medieval Moghrabi quarter to enlarge the plaza below the Wailing Wall. On the edge of the city I saw annexed land being planted with pines. Planting trees in Israel had long been a rallying image for Jews throughout the diaspora, an evocation of peaceful development that featured strongly in the information films sent out by the Jewish National Fund. They showed to Jewish clubs and schools and social groups, and idealistic Jews across the world tipped cash into the JNF's blue collection tins. But the country in whose growth the money was being invested appeared to me far from the utopia shown in these films.

Israeli society was stratified along lines of class and colour. European Askenazi Jews looked down on the Sephardis, driven from Spain by the Inquisition and living in Palestine for centuries before the advent of Zionism. Both scorned Jews from Iraq and Turkey, who in turn placed themselves above the North African Jews from Morocco, Algeria, Libya and Egypt. These groups had their own hierarchy, with those darkest-skinned and poorest – many had been forced to leave their assets behind when they had emigrated – receiving the toughest deal. At the bottom were the Yemeni Jews, brought out in a much-publicised exodus in the early 1950s and dumped in tented reception camps. Many were still there in 1968, perpetual losers in terms of housing and education. Others ended up in baking desert townships such as Dimona – its name means mirage – on the road to the Dead Sea. Each time I passed through it, Dimona's concrete tenements were lost in a dust-storm through which flitted the odd, swathed figure. Below even the Yemenis were the Israeli Arabs, descendents of the sixty-five thousand or so Muslim, Christian, Bedouin and Druse who'd been still within the borders of Israel at the end of the 1948 War.

In Haifa I'd met a group of young Israelis. One of them had an impressive collection of militaria from the recent conflict – an AK-47 bayonet, a Syrian helmet, and a broken Jordanian flare pistol which he gave to me – and another interest which I did not share. He and his friends used to go out at night to find Israeli Arabs to bash; his gang had, he said, put a couple of them in hospital. But the real target of his hatred was the Palestinians. He announced that he was looking forward to his three years of military service, when he would get a chance to shoot them.

The hard-line ideology that had produced the Deir Yassin massacre had never gone away, even though the Revisionist party led by ex-Irgun leader Menachem Begin had remained marginalized in parliamentary opposition ever since the country's first elections in 1949. Then, in the tense days leading up to the start of the 1967 war, a cross-party Government of National Unity had been formed, with Begin made a minister. Military victory gave Israel control over more than a million Palestinians – the population of the West Bank and the Gaza Strip – the majority of whom had fled into these areas from Israel as refugees in 1948. The Six-Day War had been launched to neutralise a military threat from Egypt; its escalation to include a second front on the West Bank against the Jordanians and a third against the Syrians in the north had not been foreseen. Israeli generals now feared the toll on army morale of being an occupying force and wanted to withdraw, retaining control of only the strategic Golan Heights.

But the politicians saw little reason for retreat. The Revisionists and religious right claimed that the victory had restored the lands of greater Judea to their rightful rulers, while Ben-Gurion, who'd remained opposed throughout his premiership to any coalition between Labour and the Revisionists, had since before the 1956 Suez War moved his party and government to a position that was often as hard-line and militaristic as theirs. The Government of National Unity's first post-conflict decision was to annex East Jerusalem – to restore the Wailing Wall to the heart of Zion – and there was general consensus that the outcome of the Six-Day War satisfied both those invoking divine destiny and those who talked in terms of territorial security; on Israeli State Radio the secular United Kibbutz Council was demanding that new settlements be established forthwith in the 'liberated areas'.

In this triumphalist atmosphere we were taken on a tour of the conquered lands. Near Jericho they trucked us through a refugee camp of cinderblock and plywood shacks that had until recently been occupied by eighty thousand Palestinians. It was now deserted but for abandoned dogs. Most of Jericho town's Arab population had not fled but were keeping low; the café tables under the pepper trees in the main square were patronised by Israeli soldiers, rifles by their sides, eating *falafel*. We visited the Monastery of the Rock of the Temptation, jammed into a crack on a cliff-face that housed the cave where Jesus had reputedly been propositioned by the devil. Below stretched a vista of Arabness. Robed women carried water jars on a track along the valley; a line of tiny donkeys were herded by boys with their heads swathed in *keffiyehs*. Jericho's low-domed roofs slumbered among the date palms and a haze shadowed the valley of the Jordan. This was the retreating edge of the East that had once begun at the Mediterranean coast, now strip-developed in the hybrid modern style of the State of Israel. The monastery toilet was a wooden room cantilevered out over the void, with oval holes cut in the floor. The dung of centuries formed a black crust on the rocks far below. I noticed that there was no toilet paper; a bucket of water indicated that the monks cleaned themselves in the Muslim fashion. Some of the boys straddled the holes to piss on the Arabs but the up-draft spattered their urine against the ceiling. I tossed out a handful of Israeli small change and the aluminium coins danced like fish in the column of air.

From here the truck took us eastward to the Allenby Bridge, one of the crossing points over the Jordan through which war-displaced Palestinians were gradually making their way back to their homes in the occupied West Bank. We passed a group of them, heavily laden, trudging along the roadside. An old man in a shapeless suit glanced up at us. From the back of our open truck some of the kids began to yell and jeer.

'Bush pigs! Sand kaffirs!' screamed Norm, and reached down beside his foot as though seeking a stone to throw. I was surprised at how violently his attitude offended me. In South Africa, where such behaviour was commonplace among white schoolboys, it might have passed pretty much without comment; here it seemed shocking, and I was provoked into saying something about him being a racist. This provoked a storm of abuse.

'You know what you are?' snarled Tubmann. 'You're a fucking traitor; an anti-Semite!'

A murmur spread down the truck – 'Kaplan's a fucking anti-Semite' – and fingers jabbed my chest. Far outweighing my contempt for their stupidity was my own self-loathing as I scrabbled to defend my Jewish credentials: my father had been a Mahal volunteer, an uncle had been wounded in the recent war. From under their yarmulkes Norm and Tubmann continued to regard me with unforgiving hatred.

Jewish nationalism was ascendant. In Jerusalem I'd been challenged near the Wailing Wall by aggressive young men with Brooklyn accents – members of an ultra-Orthodox religious group – holding prayer books.

'Why is your head not covered?' they had demanded, 'Are you not a Jew?' The 1967 victory had invigorated their zealotry and they were setting up fortified settlements in the occupied territories of the West Bank and Gaza Strip; one group had established itself in the centre of the Arab town of Hebron and, despite the provocative nature of this action, was receiving active support from the government. Israel appeared at the peak of its power. Moderate voices warning that the occupation would result in implacable Palestinian resistance, international condemnation and the brutalisation of the Israeli military were being ignored. Few in the country could foresee this as the beginning of its decline.

✛

I was oblivious too, young and enthralled by my own discoveries. In the north we visited the Golan Heights, jumping from boulder to boulder – in case of uncleared mines – to explore the trench systems of the Syrian defences. These had been captured in the last twenty-four hours of the Six-Day War when Egyptian and Jordanian resistance had already collapsed and it was deemed a sound strategic move to take the heights from which Syrian guns had been able to fire on the settlements along Israel's northern border.

At a kibbutz below the heights, that had been one of those targeted, every building had its counterpart underground. We saw the eating hall and its shelter, the school and its shelter, the children's crèche and its shelter. The sick-bay was complemented by an underground dressing station, buried beneath the ramparts of the kibbutz defences and reached via a web of trenches. Daylight through the dug-out entrance illuminated a raised bench along the walls on which casualties could be laid. Primus lamps hung ready on hooks and shelves were stacked with satchels of khaki canvas, each bearing a painted red cross. I looked inside one of them at the array of packaged gauze and dressings, scissors, clamps, intravenous fluid packs and ampoules of drugs. This was the thing my father did, the special knowledge that made him a doctor. And in a premonitory glimpse I saw the truth at the heart of the practice of medicine: that there was no mystery, that learning and skill turned these ordered bits of equipment into the means of stopping bleeding and bringing together shattered tissue to make a greater order, to save a life.

There'd been many threats to the survival of those who'd founded these early kibbutzes in the north. The settlers fought regular skirmishes with the inhabitants of nearby Arab villages. In the winters they were in danger of being flooded by the rains, in spring by snow-melt off the slopes of Mount Hermon. During summer the area swarmed with malarial mosquitoes, causing constant illness. In 1943 my dad, on leave from his field hospital in Egypt, had come to this part of Palestine. Once out of uniform he'd made contact with the Haganah, who took him to meet the committee running these border kibbutzes. He was bearing gifts. The first was a pistol, a war souvenir acquired from one of the patients under his care at the field hospital. The second present was of far greater value: two thousand tablets of the synthetic anti-malarial Atabrin, German army medical supplies captured from retreating Axis forces after the Battle of El- Alamein.

Now here I was in one of those kibbutzes he had helped, in a country which – as a volunteer in Israel's War of Independence – he had helped to bring into being. It was late at night and we were sitting in the community centre, watching a squad of paratroopers getting ready for a cross-border raid into southern Lebanon. The young men joked as they prepared their equipment. One played the guitar, another stripped and reassembled his Uzi submachine gun with lightning fingers before our admiring gaze. The order came for them to go. Shrugging on their equipment, they stood while their officer inspected every man. Now they checked their weapons. Each soldier, before he stuck the clip back into his Uzi, carried out the same gesture, like a good luck ritual: tapping the magazine – *clonk clonk* – against his helmet to make sure the rounds would feed properly. Then they filed out, climbing onto the blacked-out trucks that would take them to the infiltration point in Mount Hermon's foothills.

Most of the kids in our group went to bed, but I and a young German kibbutznik climbed to the top of the water tower. We sat on the concrete roof of the tank, shivering in the cold and staring into the darkness to the north. He gave me a cigarette. An amateur, I choked and coughed until, feeling foolish, I cupped it in my palm, relishing the small ember of warmth. From the hills came a faint crackle of noise. '*Tat-miklah*' – submachine gun – said the German boy.

There was another sound like distant balloons popping. Above the horizon a parachute flare ignited and dropped slowly, leaving a flickering glow that silhouetted the hillsides. From the border, perhaps a mile north of the kibbutz, a heavy machine gun began firing, sending red tracers in a long, curving parabola. It continued for a long time, joined sometimes by another weapon further west, covering the soldiers' withdrawal. Beside me the German boy lit another cigarette. He sucked the smoke down hard and serious, like a man.

✛

I felt I was growing up. At a dance one night at a kibbutz on the coast I met an Israeli girl. Tova had blond hair cut short and a corduroy work-shirt. After I'd danced with her awhile in uncoordinated awkwardness, she proposed that we go for a walk. Outside, she took my hand. I was astonished, for in my limited experience it had been myself, the ardent, clumsy boy, who had tried to take the lead, only to fail in the face of female prudery or plain good sense. How could this girl – walking me through the streets of the settlement towards the beach – not have the same reaction? Trying to reassure her of my harmlessness, I talked and talked, seemingly unable to get to the end of whatever I had started to say. Some soldiers at the perimeter fence asked where we were going. Telling them to mind their business, Tova led me into the darkness. One of the men winked at me. In the dunes I stumbled on the salt-grass but she pulled me effortlessly upright, and I realised that she was much stronger than I was. Then she kissed me and, undoing a button on her shirt, guided my hand onto her breast.

The next evening, reunited with my group from Sde Boqer, we travelled through Tel Aviv. Above the sky-line stood a red neon sign. It consisted of the Hebrew letters *kuf, nun, tet* and was an advertisement for Kent cigarettes, but in demotic, vowel-less Hebrew it also spelled cunt, which was considered a joke of huge sophistication by the blokes in the group. I felt entirely superior to them, though in fact I knew little more about sex than I had before I met Tova; the sensation of her tongue against mine and the way her nipple had teased my palm had been so overwhelming that I retained only the most ethereal impression of her smooth, resilient body. I hadn't even any visual memories to go on, for everything had happened in the dark, but I felt I'd glimpsed a sort of ecstasy that life could sometimes be perfect. Back at Sde Boqer I wrote to Tova in my best Hebrew, painstakingly inscribed on one of the utilitarian white-on-both-sides Israeli postcards, asking her to come and visit me on the kibbutz. Her reply was hand-delivered by a soldier passing through Sde Boqer on his way south. Written in English and sealed in a tiny envelope, she informed me that her boyfriend was returning soon from the Sinai where he had been on military service. Coming to see me would be complicated. She knew, she said, that I'd understand.

Our Hebrew classes resumed, while I thought only of Tova and all the things, half comprehended, that we hadn't done. The tedium of the lessons was broken a couple of times by a Mirage jet-fighter whose pilot had a girlfriend on our kibbutz. He would bring his plane low over the desert from the west, howl above our heads and climb into a half roll before diving out of sight, only to reappear over the lip of the gorge and return like a bullet, his exhaust buffeting the prefab classrooms. We stood outside and cheered, our hands over our ears as the aircraft came over again and again at rooftop height, strumming the kinked washing-lines strung across the yard. Cursing, the kibbutz administrator would order us back to our lessons and storm off to call the air force base. I knew exactly what that pilot was feeling.

◎

It was a relief when an opportunity came to visit the Sinai. Some soldiers from the kibbutz were using their leave to see this newly conquered territory and would escort our group. The kibbutz nurse joined the party, which was led by David the archaeologist, an Uzi on his shoulder. We set off in two Bedford trucks, fitted out with wooden benches as troop carriers. The posts of their awnings each bore a rifle in a canvas case. We travelled the short distance – around thirty miles – to the old Egyptian border and then swung south onto a dirt track that wound between dry hills. Nightfall found us grinding along a sand-bottomed wadi. The vehicles stopped and in their headlights we sorted out our camp, choosing sleeping places between the boulders. A meal of cucumbers, cheese and flat bread was distributed, guards posted, and we went to sleep.

At four A.M. David shook us awake. Shivering, I pulled on my boots and leather coat, turning up its collar, and joined the few who had bothered to rouse themselves. We started up a narrow notch in the wadi's side, climbing in the dark, scrabbling up the steeper sections with the help of David's long arm. Gradually it became possible to see some detail and I realised the sky was lightening; as we reached the crest, a rich band of pink was building along the horizon. We found we were standing on smooth stone, a paved platform among the rocks from which tall stelae – their tips beginning to be bathed in orange light – stuck skyward above our heads. The place was the location of an ancient Egyptian opal mine, the hieroglyphs on the stones, translated by David, proclaiming this as a temple to the god Horus. Even the dimmest of us was struck with wonder.

After breakfast we continued westwards on a track that cut through empty desert. Sometimes it followed a faint depression, marked by sparse scrub as the bed of a watercourse. Israeli army trucks passed us, heading the other way with waves and hooting. Occasionally a spot in the distance would draw near through the heat-shimmer and resolve itself into a crossroads, marked by an oil barrel supporting a post that carried military unit signs and a water tank for topping up army radiators. A wind blew in our faces like the breath from an oven. A couple of hours later objects began to appear along the wayside, studding the ground. They were boots, thousands of them scattered across the desert, each the start of a small dune that had formed in its lee.

At the time of the Six-Day War the pictures of these abandoned boots had appeared in newspapers and magazines around the world. I remembered the plummy voice of the announcer on MovieTone News describing how they had been thrown aside in terror by the Egyptian soldiers so they could run faster to their homes across the Canal. Looking at the wasteland around us, I commented that it seemed strange that they would choose to flee barefoot across the baking sand. Avi, one of the soldiers, explained that Egyptian prisoners had been ordered to take off their boots by the Israelis in order to stop them from trying to escape; the international newsmen had all preferred the simplistic symbol of ignominious Arab defeat.

The road we were following began to wind upward through a range of hills. This was the Mitla Pass, the last barrier before the Canal lying thirty miles westward. The geographic features that made the pass a natural defensive position also made it a trap, for the retreating Egyptian forces, funnelled into its narrow confines, had been smashed from the air by Israeli planes. A jam of broken trucks and field guns blocked the road and spread across the blackened sand. The desert was carpeted with skeins of machine-gun belts and live artillery shells flung from shattered transports. We wound among them, following the ruts of other vehicles that had found a route through this vast still-life. Israeli bombs had wrought spectacular distortions. Trucks were buckled so that only their front and rear bumpers touched the ground, and armoured half-tracks had been ruptured by explosions that had forced their sides out like metal sails, perforated by a thousand holes through which the sunlight flared.

We edged past a column of tanks, hatches open and guns frozen at odd angles. At the top of the pass we dismounted and walked up a low ridge to where more armour stood, half dug into the earth.

I climbed the side of a tank and lowered myself down into the gunner's position. Inside it smelled of heated metal and something rancid, like a distillation of old sweat. The prism of the periscope was smeared with a waxy substance that got under my fingernails. On the side of the gun breach was a metal plate with printing on it, that I tried to pry off with my penknife. Then I noticed on the steel shelf before me a row of human teeth. I tapped them with my knife but they appeared fused to the metal. The smell was overpowering and I felt that I would vomit, so I pulled myself out of the turret and back into the light. Some boys had found a line of toes sticking out of the drifted sand, the skin shrunk and mummified. Before they could disturb the body David ordered us back to the trucks.

Dunes had encroached across the road beyond the pass, so that our wheels bucked and ploughed over the hummocks. Closer to the canal were high berms of bulldozed sand, sheltering tents and vehicle parks. Avi pointed out a smudge in the distance above the heat-ripple: the roofs of the town of Suez. A military police jeep came bouncing towards us over the criss-cross of wheel-tracks, the man beside the driver hanging on with one hand as he gesticulated to us with the other. 'Slowly, slowly,' he yelled as he drew up alongside. 'You're raising dust! Their gunners will see it!' The forward positions were too dangerous for us to approach, he explained; shelling the previous day had killed ten Israeli soldiers. He advised us to turn south.

The route stretched across a plain as white as salt that threw back a blinding glare, and we drew the folds of our *keffiyehs* that we'd learned to wear Arab-style into slits across our eyes, covering our mouths against the scorching wind. The road converged with the coastline and the sea appeared, a blue so deep that I imagined I could feel its coolness bathing my retinas. For some time we skirted the water's edge until the trucks stopped in a grove of date-palms. The place was a fishing village, quite deserted. I stepped through fallen palm fronds onto the beach. A line of dhows was pulled up on the sand. Small waves rapped at the shingle below their rudders and a steady wind droned in the rigging and rattled the halyards against the masts. Houses along the single street stood open, doors banging in the dust-eddies that pirouetted across the sand.

'Don't touch anything,' shouted David, but the kids were already disappearing among the buildings.

I entered the nearest, a place with walls of ochre mud. Shoes were lined inside the entrance: a pair of men's lace-ups cracked across the instep, low-heeled slippers and some children's sandals. Light came in as a window shutter swung open and closed. Sand rasped underfoot. On a table were plates and glasses covered with dust, and a brick-hard loaf of bread. The wooden shelf held volumes in Arabic and some school exercise books. A trail of clothes lay across the floor, dropped in the haste of flight or rejected by looters.

'Poor people's house,' said David, looking around. From outside came shouts and breaking glass. He ran out, cursing.

'We found a box of hand-grenades,' yelled one of the boys. 'These are the houses of terrorists!'

'Just leave them alone,' ordered David. 'We'll tell the army about the grenades. Get back on the trucks.'

'They should never be allowed back,' Tubmann said as we remounted. 'Fucking terrorists.'

Turning inland, the road began to twist along the side of black mountains. It skirted a valley, revealing an unexpected swathe of green: an oasis, the first one I'd seen, with palms and shade and tiny stone-walled fields. A glint of water showed beneath the clustered palms but beyond their fringe the bare sand began abruptly. Our route wound higher among the peaks. On either side were the mouths of shafts and tunnels cut into the rock. The trucks crept up a track that clung to the side of a cliff, turned in through a great, dark cavern, the engine-noise battering off the walls, and emerged abruptly into daylight. Ahead stood buildings – workshops, storerooms and a small mosque – the offices of a manganese mine, perched on a platform hewn from the edge of the mountain's summit. From the terrace in front of the manager's house we could see over burned-looking peaks and the deep blue of the Gulf of Suez to the far side, a pale reddish coastline that was the Egyptian shore.

Forsaking the view, I joined Morris and Ishie to explore the cavern through which we'd arrived. Its walls and roof were lost in darkness. Chains hung down from above and somewhere water splashed, echoingly. Away to one side was a small square of daylight. We walked towards it, stumbling on the ties of a narrow-gauge rail track. Ore-trucks stood at intervals along it. The track emerged through the opening into bright sunlight, where an ore-truck waited on a siding, its bucket piled with rock. A brake-bar prevented it passing onward along the rails which traversed the cliff-side. At its end the track looped out over the precipice on timber props, incorporating a mechanism designed to tip the bucket as each truck passed over it, for a pinnacle of crushed rock began a hundred feet below and spread downwards to disappear in the depths of the gorge. Ishie shifted the brake and the heavy truck groaned, inching forward on the track.

Tubmann and Norm had appeared, flanked by the Aarons. 'Let's get another one,' proposed Tubmann, and we went back into the darkness and put our shoulders to the next truck. With our combined weight it began to move forward slowly, then more easily. Reaching daylight, it thudded over the points to strike with a clash of couplings against the truck already there. Tubmann clapped me on the shoulder. 'More, man, more,' he said excitedly; it seemed I was one of the group. Working together, we repeated the process until four ore-trucks stood in line. Then Ishie threw the bar up and they were off, at a walk and then a trot and then, with a rocking rumble that shook the tracks, a gallop of iron and stone. At the loop they did not falter but sailed out into the void in a plunging train, shedding rocks and dust. They hit the peak of the tailings pile and the noise began, a booming, clanging avalanche down the rubble slopes that echoed through the gorge, which boiled a mounting cloud of dust. We ran silently away, exhilarated by the volume of destruction. I saw in that instant how seductive it was to be a destroyer; to dynamite buildings, perpetrate massacres, to know the intoxicating freedom from restraint. We emerged from the cavern, the echoes of rockfalls still rumbling, and straight into David's rage.

'Its' just fucking Gyppo crap,' objected Tubmann, scornfully.

I stood at the edge of the group, saying nothing. David glared at me. I wished I'd stayed an anti-Semite.

The road took us inland through ranges of mountains. That evening the desert delivered up its first humans. We had stopped in a wadi to set up our camp and were discussing unenthusiastically what fare would be served up for dinner, when there came the clink of stones and a herd of goats streamed by in the dusk like smoke, dividing and merging along invisible tracks on the wadi's rocky side. Two figures followed them, flitting across the slope. David called out in Arabic and the men descended cautiously. Over their burnouses they wore army greatcoats, perhaps discarded by retreating Egyptians the year before. I noticed that one of our soldiers had slipped a rifle from its cover and was standing behind a truck with it near to hand. David talked with the Bedouin for a while and handed out some tins of food and cigarettes. Our nurse added aspirin and vitamin tablets for their children. Then the men were gone, leaping from rock to rock after their departed goats. That night guards were posted again – we had become slack about this discipline since we'd entered the desert – and they changed shifts through the night, stamping around atop the truck's metal cabs and keeping everyone awake with intermittent shouts of alarm. David had the rest of the rifles removed from their canvas sleeves and loaded for use, but wisely refused to issue them.

Our journey the next morning continued along a riverbed, up and over a long, stepped ridge and then along another wadi until we joined a visible road: the old pilgrim route to Santa Katerina Monastery at the bottom of Jebel Musa, Mount Sinai. The monastery, founded in the sixth century, had until recently prohibited access to women. Male visitors and food (including male livestock) had been admitted by basket, lowered from a hoist incorporated in one of the defensive overhangs atop its surrounding wall that also allowed monks to drop missiles on the heads of attackers. Only in the last couple of years had a postern gate been cut through the wall's base and, stiff from the day's driving, we shuffled through it into a courtyard of palms and oleanders and dusty red flowers. I think a fountain played, though this may have been in my imagination, for my senses were so overwhelmed by the rich foliage that I remembered little of the monastery but a scent of lemon trees and an alley between stone walls that framed dark cypresses along the columned front of a basilica.

Near sunset we were guided by an English-speaking lay brother to the place where we would sleep. He sat in the truck's cab to show the route past stony fields, identifying the sites where monks had been murdered over the centuries by marauding nomads. The track entered a wide, arid valley. At its far end stood a speck of white, and as our vehicles drove slowly over the ribbed riverbed it resolved into a house, its front luminous in the fading light. The building was another shock to my parched senses, for the sheer ordinariness of the structure – double-storied, with an attic window in the gable – gave it a pleasant air of welcome. I asked our guide what it was.

'American house,' he said disinterestedly, 'build by American mission for visiting pilgrims. We stop here,' and he directed the trucks towards an inlet in the valley wall. We were unloaded and began to make camp, while one vehicle set off back along the track to take him back to the monastery.

The truck returned and manoeuvred back and forth to park tail-on to the rocks, the gap between it and its fellow forming a laager in which we would sleep. I climbed a little way up the valley side and looked along it. A hundred yards away black goat's-wool Bedouin tents were pitched on the sand, and their camels, cruelly hobbled against flight with a rope that kept one forefoot hoisted high in front, hopped from shrub to shrub along the slopes. Beyond them stood the house on a little rise above the valley floor, and though the sky was tipping into darkness it continued to gather and reflect back a residual light until it too passed into obscurity. No lights appeared in its windows.

On the tail-flaps of the trucks, slung horizontal to serve as tables, those of us assigned to kitchen duties began opening drums of baked beans and sawing rubbery bread. Big gas cookers flared blue under the pots. I stirred the mess, staying close to their heat, for the night already seemed to be the coldest we had experienced. After we had eaten and mopped our plates with bread, stacking them unwashed in their crates, a group of us set off into the darkness to find firewood. A mysterious line of bobbing shapes among the rocks resolved into the naked bottoms of the girls of our party, pissing in a row; as we passed they squealed and jumped, pulling up their jeans. The mountains stood black against a vault of stars, from which descended a bone-aching chill that cut through the fleece lining of my coat. Even better than firewood, I thought, was the possibility that the house might offer shelter against the freezing night.

We skirted the Bedouin tents, marked by small orange fires – not unlike the light-bulb in that diorama at the Desert Museum in Sde Boqer – and the yapping of dogs. In the darkness the hobbled camels stumbled over the rocks, groaning like arthritics. As we approached the house I could see that it was made of solid clapboard. So strong was my conviction that the place must be in use that it seemed inconceivable that the front door would be standing open; or rather, that there was no door at all, for I stepped through the entrance and found myself standing on the desert, with beyond the dark rise of the mountainside. All that remained of the American house was the façade. The rest – back, sides, floorboards and internal partitions – had been unpicked over the years and taken for firewood by the nomads and caravans passing through this barren valley. Even the last struts of two-by-four that braced the corners had been whittled away for kindling by sharp blades. The cold gripped me harder.

Back at the trucks we snapped twigs from the tough desert bushes that had been crushed by our tyres and, breaking up a food crate, managed to get a blaze going. We stood over it, thrusting our hands into the flames to warm them. Gradually the others went to their sleeping places but I stayed up, feeding the fire with whatever I could find that might burn. On a further foraging trip I stole some cakes of goat-dung from a stone ledge where they'd been set to dry. I knew the enormity of my transgression – in a place so bare even shit had value – but I was too cold to care. I placed them on the coals and watched them catch and glow, pulsating in the night wind. I hunched as close as I could to the warmth, wrapped around it so none should escape. The burning dung gave off an animal reek that soaked into my clothes. The last embers faded. I went to the hollow where I had left my sleeping bag and climbed inside, feeling the hoarded heat flow away from me into the freezing ground.

It was still dark when they roused us. I had spent the last hours in a shivering knot and found it difficult to uncurl my limbs. Mugs of *mitz* and sweet biscuits were handed out. Then we boarded the trucks and were carried back along the track to begin the ascent of Jebel Musa. At the start of the pilgrim's way we dismounted and Galli the cook handed out breakfast, a plastic bag containing a leathery orange and two slices of bread glued together with a spread of alum-like tartness. Our path was a camel track that rose between the boulders, wide enough for two or three to walk abreast. I trudged upwards amidst a group of my friends. There was something wrong with my perceptions. Ivan was joking with Zimmy; their chatter seemed weighed with significance yet at the same time infuriated me with its lack of logic. I tried to interject but my words produced only strange looks. My legs felt extraordinarily heavy, my body weightless. The wind seemed to blow through me, vibrating the ice in my bones.

The predawn sky paled as we climbed. I tripped, the fall bringing my face within inches of a bulge of rock. In the half-light it resembled exactly the glutinous semolina they sometimes fed us for breakfast at the kibbutz and I licked it like a dog. A couple of the boys pulled me to my feet.

'Kaplan's gone mad,' they said. Ivan asked me if I was okay. I laughed and forged onward through a landscape that coruscated with impossible light, as though from the dung-smoke I had inhaled some profound hallucinogen. We reached the summit just before the sun, gathering on a flat place at a chapel whose white walls radiated a shimmering aura. Globular ranges of mountains still lay in shadow except for the peak of Jebel Katerina to the south which glowed red, the shrine on its top like a flame. Heated by the climb, people around me began to shed their jackets. Despite my exertions I had never been colder and I begged them for their garments, putting them on layer and layer over my leather coat. I tore open my breakfast bag and sucked at the orange, its juice seeming to evaporate at once in my desiccated mouth.

During the descent, deafened by the pulse in my ears, insulated from the environment by my cocoon of clothing, I staggered oblivious down the path. At one point I stepped off the ledge and fell ten feet onto a lower traverse, but I felt nothing, not even the shock of landing. We were returning along a different route of steep stone steps that led down to the monastery. It lay far below us, a rectangle of ochre battlements enclosing roofs and belfries among the trees, unreal and unreachable. Eventually, half steered, half supported, I reached the bottom of the mountain and was led to the foot of the monastery wall, where I plunged immediately into a deep and pathological sleep interrupted by bouts of shivering so violent that my spine was bruised as it banged against the ground. During one of these awakenings I noticed that the sunlight had receded and that I lay in a band of grey shadow. The wall, the mountains beyond, even the people around me seemed bleached of life.

Then I was in one of the trucks, stretched out in my sleeping bag along a bench. We were driving, but I couldn't distinguish between the shivers that racked me and the hammering of the tyres over the stones. Sometimes the nurse bent over me, looking worried, while I argued with a second self whose body stretched into limitless distance while its limbs lay on mine, crushing me with a weight of pain. In my delirium we travelled through a desert of rocks so sharp their points were invisible, so fine that they crumbled to crystals the instant they pierced my skin, which itched all over as though inoculated with powdered glass. I took refuge in a landscape of green bluffs and bays filled with boats, but the land shuddered and the water surged away, leaving the yachts canted on the sand, and returned as a black, towering wave that rushed upon me. When I shouted, trying to swim, people shook me. I could tell that they were concerned, for in a period of clarity I understood the nurse asking me whether I had a thousand dollars to pay for a helicopter that was standing by to come and fly me to a hospital in Tel Aviv. I said no, for I knew I had to keep my two hundred in traveller's cheques cached against an emergency; then the embrace of my fever pulled me away under the surface of consciousness to wrestle anew.

When I awoke, drained but lucid, two days had passed and we were heading south on the coast road that led to the tip of the Sinai. Sometime in the last twenty-four hours the bench opposite had become occupied by another patient, a dark-haired girl named

Becky. She lay there mute, apparently in retreat from some great shock. The nurse seemed relieved to have me back, to share the diagnostic responsibility.

'I don't know what's happened to her,' she confided to me, the proxy doctor. 'A big fright of some kind. Maybe someone tried to rape her.'

I looked at the figure on the other bench, her eyelids trembling. Suddenly I felt the recipient of too much knowledge. I did not want the thought that someone could have forced violence on this fragile person.

'Becky,' I said, close to her ear, 'it's okay, you're safe now,' watching her profile for a response. I arranged my *keffiyeh* to shield her face from the sun and poured mugs of water for the nurse, who held them to her lips.

My health continued to improve and at Sharm el Sheikh – below the abandoned Egyptian gun positions, still sown with mines – I lay on the beach in the sun, feeling its warmth dispel the last of my illness. As we travelled north up the edge of the Gulf of Aqaba I was well enough to float over the coral reefs and, with a diving-mask borrowed from Avi, to look down on flashing swarms of fish. Becky had surfaced from her state of withdrawal and rejoined her friends, without ever revealing what had been the cause of her brief derangement. Until recently she had not stood out in any way from the group; now I saw her in a special light, through the responsibility I'd assumed in helping to look after her.

On our return to the kibbutz we two were considered still to be sick – neither of us had had our conditions diagnosed – and we were put in the sick-bay for blood tests. These were uncomfortable, for the medic considered gentleness to be analogous to softness. His regime of vitamin injections I refused absolutely – as the son of a doctor I was acknowledged this right – but I was expected instead to assume responsibility for some tasks. I carried buckets of vomit and mopped the floor and accompanied the nurse on her morning round, bearing the steel tray with syringes for the other patients. Becky took her treatment with resignation, rolling onto her front and gasping at the pain of the injection. I looked away, my teeth clenched in sympathy. In the afternoons she was visited by her friends; one, a red-head named Diane, would always greet me with an ironic, 'How's the doctor?'

They'd whisper around Becky's bed, glancing at me and giggling. The boys that were my friends were infrequent visitors, dropping by to bring dog-eared novels passed around for their sexual content. These gave me powerful erections but no advice on how to start a conversation with Becky's friends. After a week, the blood tests having shown no abnormalities, I was discharged with a diagnosis of 'desert fever' – probably from an insect bite – and returned to my quarters.

Autumn had come while I'd been an inpatient, bringing a wind that moaned through the concrete houses. At night it was too cold to sleep on the roofs, so those wanting to avoid guard duty had to find other places to hide, except that a peculiar *cafard* now gripped us; the duty officer bursting into our rooms at midnight with shouts of '*Kvutz! kvutz!*' – Jump! Jump! – was as likely to be met with cries of 'Fuck off!' as with obedience. One day, when the wind was silent and a stillness sat on the desert, they packed us off on a bus to refresh our martial spirit. The destination was a military airfield tucked away in the depths of the Negev. South of Beersheba the bus swung off the main road onto a dirt track through a wadi. After several bends between high banks the track became tarred with a security fence and gate, and a guard post where we were stopped by soldiers. Cameras, we were told, were forbidden beyond this point and must be sealed in bags; any that were seen would be confiscated. Tubmann and Norm, awoken to officiousness by the issuing of orders, went round checking that everyone obeyed. An officer boarded the bus and guided us through the base to a parking area, where we climbed down.

The occasion was a military air display. The US Senate, under vigorous lobbying, had agreed to supply Israel with its top-line fighter, the F-16 Phantom, and the first shipments of the aircraft had recently arrived. Checked and put through their trials, they were now ready to be exhibited before a chosen audience of Israeli brass and American-Jewish civic leaders whose representation had got the deal through; the latter had combined their visit with a holiday in the Holy Land, and family groups strolled around the airfield in

Bermuda shorts and sun hats as though at Disneyland. We youthful visitors from the diaspora, expected sources of future support for Israel, had been invited too. A buffet had been laid out under a camouflage-net pergola, and we swooped on the little sandwiches like ravenous crows.

The event was also an arms fair for Israeli Military Industries to show off its expertise; the upgrading of French- and US-supplied helicopters and ground attack planes with Israeli avionics and weapons systems. Aircraft were parked in front of the control tower, their bombs, rockets ands cannon shells laid in neat patterns under their wings. Stern soldiers, weapons slung, kept the tourists behind rope barriers that prevented them touching these menacing icons, while uniformed attachés from some of the countries which Israel armed – Stroessner's Paraguay, Mobutu's Congo, Somoza's Nicaragua – inspected the hardware close up. Then the loudspeakers crackled, inviting us to take our seats for the display. Banks of seating had been erected on the runway edge, the scaffolding trimmed with white and blue bunting, and we clambered up to the top row with our hands over our ears as a pair of the new jets took off, their afterburners roaring.

Overhead they cavorted in mock-combat attacks and barrel-rolls, then climbed high to disappear in the sky's glare. There was a silence, then the buzz of voices; military escorts were pointing out to their guests a line of tanks and trucks that stood a thousand yards from us across the desert sand. On the horizon a dot appeared. It approached with a deafening shriek and racketed overhead. At the same instant the row of vehicles disappeared in a curtain of flashes and spinning fragments. The jet had flipped to one side and now the other dived in, firing rockets that trailed a white streak as they closed on the target. More pieces flew and something started burning, pumping up black smoke that was instantly shredded by the first plane as it raked the line of vehicles from end to end with its cannons. By now the grandstand was rocking with fervour, the visitors on their feet screaming and cheering. The lead jet dropped cluster bombs that flayed the surface of the desert so that it jumped and smoked. Then the aircraft returned together, wingtip to wingtip, low above the sand. From their bellies tumbled long cylinders that bounced end on end along the column. The napalm ignited with a thud – the shock-wave struck our faces seconds later – and fire formed a writhing wall where the vehicles had been. Weapons like these had wrought such destruction on the Egyptian soldiers in the Mitla Pass. I realised that this was what modern war meant: devastating wounds; scant heroism; indeed, hardly any chance of surviving that obliterating inferno.

✛

Our service done, we flew back to South Africa and I shared a bottle of sticky liqueur with Ishie and Morris in the back row of the plane. Later, when the cabin was in darkness, Becky walked by. I stood and spoke her name. She stared at me, her mouth slightly open, and I saw that there was nothing to say: she felt no bond between us, but I'd gained something from her that would endure, despite the fact that we would never see each other again. I stepped back and she walked past me up the aisle. We landed in Johannesburg and the customs man looked in my suitcase. I watched him flick through the bullet shells, rusted links of machine-gun belt, the twisted flare pistol; the husks of old wars. His hand rooted in a desultory fashion beneath my folded leather coat. I was acutely aware of the proscribed publications – pornographic and political – hidden inside it. I'd left home barely aware, not questioning the strangeness of how we lived in South Africa or whether I believed in Zionism. Somewhere during my time away a part of my youth had passed; a romance, a trust in the rightness of things. Now all I knew was who I was not.

My father had visited Palestine with pistol and Atabrin tablets, life-saving gifts for the Jewish pioneers. As a result of his surgical work during the War of Independence there were probably a lot of ex-Haganah men walking on two legs that might have been amputees if he hadn't volunteered. He was back in Israel during the October War of 1973, treating wounded soldiers at the Hadassah Hospital in Jerusalem after an Egyptian offensive across the Suez Canal had inflicted heavy losses on the not-so-invincible Israelis. It took Israel's 1982 invasion of Lebanon – ordered by the ex-Irgun leader Menachem Begin, who'd become prime minister – to shake his support for the country, when Israeli forces stood back while their Phalangist Christian allies massacred some two thousand Palestinian civilians in the Sabra and Chatilla refugee camps. His last visit to Israel was with my mother in 1998 for the ceremonies commemorating the fiftieth anniversary of the founding of the state, when they joined the survivors of the five thousand Mahal overseas volunteers who had come in 1948 to serve the cause of Israel's independence. I envy him that connectedness. Since then the country has built a wall around itself, in the largest infrastructure project it has ever undertaken. I have not returned.

3

Morbid Anatomy

With the end of that journey it felt as though another had begun, into a place of complexity. Coming home to the welcoming family barbeque on our terrace overlooking Durban Bay, I discovered that my stomach had shrunk; it rebelled ascetically against the large steak which I would previously have ingested comfortably and now blew up my belly after three mouthfuls. The view seemed too lush, our lives too rich. After distributing the gifts I had brought for my family – a Persian miniature on ivory in the traditional style, by an artist whose work my father collected; a brooch for my mother in the form of a spray of silver that looked like the leafless desert shrubs, things, original and not, for my brothers and sister – I went into the kitchen to hand out the presents I had for the other people who made up our household.

Our cook, a middle-aged Xhosa woman who was a follower of one of the African Zionist churches, received the items on the shopping list of devotional objects she'd requested. For Peter, the gardener and handyman, I had one of those 'souvenir of Jerusalem' replica Arab daggers in gilt base-metal, with a loop of chain on the scabbard to hang it on a wall.

Peter drew the blade and ran his finger along the edge. 'Needs sharpening,' he said.

I explained that the thing was purely ornamental. From his expression it was clear that he couldn't see the point of such a useless object, and frankly, neither did I. Peter had no observable religion. He was a tough, muscular Zulu of the Luthuli Clan, whose head, Chief Albert Luthuli, had in 1961 been awarded the Nobel Peace Prize for his non-violent leadership of the ANC in the face of extreme government provocation that included the Sharpeville shootings. Peter knew about the honour but spoke little of politics; he was an ex-boxer with a shaved head and fists like rocks, and he ducked low behind his hands and showed me how to protect my head and lead with my left.

He'd been my teacher in many things, passing on to me the skills acquired during his rural Zululand childhood of how to build intricate bird snares with trip-bar and noose. When I brought home an antique rifle – a Martini-Henry, the pattern that the British army had used in the Zulu War in 1879 – Peter had handled it confidently, familiar with the obsolete mechanism of loading-lever and dropping breach.

'The best kind of gun,' he said, and told me an uncle had owned one which Peter had used to hunt when he was a boy. I wondered if it was one of the weapons captured from the British in their great defeat at Isandhlwana, before the invading army had returned, greatly reinforced, with Gatling guns and cannon to cut down the Zulu regiments and subjugate their nation.

Peter liked strong drink and rum-and-maple tobacco rolled into newspaper, which he smoked on the cement steps outside his quarters, and he let me try a little of both. Periodically he would go missing and have to be collected from jail; he'd return hung-over but dignified, blood crusted at his nostrils where he'd been beaten by the cops. I only saw him once lose his composure. One afternoon, formal in his khaki uniform, he handed me a piece of paper. The number written on it, he said, was that of a white *baas* who had the details of his sister's death the day before in a tractor accident, and he asked if I would call it for him. I looked at the number, which had too many digits for a local phone and no prefix to indicate a distant exchange, and started dialling every permutation I could think of. Each was unsuccessful. As I hung up call after call, Peter sank gradually to a sitting position against the wall, his head back, weeping brokenly.

Having been years in our employ, he announced himself abruptly done with domestic work and went back to hard labour as a gardener for the Durban municipality. Eight months later we heard that he'd been killed, working in a city park, by a falling tree. The news reached us in an indefinable way, impossible to verify or date.

The cook had heard it from someone who was told it by a woman who had heard it from someone else. It was supposed to have happened many weeks before, though there was also another story that he'd died of something different, in another place. This void of communication – between our family and these people who had lived with us for years, yet remained strangers whose homes we would never visit and couldn't imagine – seemed grotesque, yet prior to going to Israel I had been largely oblivious to it.

I'd returned restless, my perceptions shaken, troubled by the inequities that seemed to underlie human interaction. I discussed this with my closest friends, George and Rob and Greg, on hiking trips across the old Anglo-Boer War battlefields. The softest sleeping-places were in grave enclosures where the goats couldn't crop the grass, and we'd rest beneath the stars beside the Unknown British Soldier and the Twelve Brave Burghers Buried Here. Three of us identified with the English; tall, blond, bush-wise Greg, whose father was a boiler-maker on the railways, was the Boer. He could tell the time by the sun, hit what he shot at, draw animals and aircraft perfect in every detail with never an erasure and hoped to be a pilot. Rob and George would do intellectual things, probably become doctors like their parents. It felt, at that youthful time, that I could have thrown myself into whatever chance might put my way. 'Life is Short,' instructed the Liar Dice manual, 'the Art long, Judgement difficult, Experience fallacious and the Occasion fleeting.'

At school I was a trouble-maker, regularly flogged and once briefly expelled for 'calculated insubordination', at loggerheads with Ivan the Intelligent, who'd been with me in Israel and now became a prefect. Demure and well-brought-up, my female classmates appeared already to be model housewives rather than potential partners in passion. None had a notion of Tova's sensuality, and my sexual dreams remained as insubstantial as the dreamy recollections of that encounter. Living in a medical household, I knew more about the theory than many of my school-friends. There was scant opportunity to learn; in South Africa the Calvinist Dutch Reformed Church dictated the Christian National syllabus, in which sex education did not feature. Neither did nipples and nudity, which were censored from films, along with any scenes containing suggestive dialogue. Even with the sexual content excised, films were additionally age-restricted – four to eighteen, four to twenty-one – so that when we succeeded in getting into these forbidden screenings, the message they conveyed was that adulthood was an enigma of jump-cut narrative and elliptical communication.

I met Peta at a party in a friend's house in the woody suburb of Westville. We kissed in the darkened garden while night-insects trilled and the family dog splashed about in the swimming pool to cool itself in the tepid water. It was at this same friend's house that we consummated our throat-pounding desire one weekend afternoon, in the garden studio of his artist mother. Our lovemaking was incompetently exquisite. We used a condom – less for contraception than because it appeared the adult thing to do – and even this banal impediment seemed suffused with erotic import. After I'd had my orgasm (I had entirely impractical ideas about how to help with hers) and we'd untangled ourselves from our complicated embrace, I tied a knot in the condom and dropped it down between the side of the bed and the wall, intending to retrieve it after a post-coital rest. From under the bed came a resonant gulp. Electrified, we stuck our heads under the bed to find the dog, blinking foolishly. The condom was gone.

We had joined our host's family for tea at the poolside when the dog appeared. It approached in abject fashion, stopping now and then to retch into the flower-beds. Then it slumped on the patio at our feet, gazing up at us with a reproachful expression and hiccupping loudly. I had a nightmare vision of it regurgitating the condom, immaculate and identifiable, on the paving, but after a while it wandered off. Though we trailed it for the rest of the day and into the evening, the dog kept down his dinner, to deposit it eventually in some remote corner where I hoped it would never be found.

✪

Now in my final year of school, I was full of unformed desires: to alleviate and redress, to vanquish and save, to travel in places where the currencies of exchange were the Atabrin or the gun. I wanted to enfilade death from both flanks. In such a campaign luck and bluff couldn't be relied on; it would be necessary to have skills. For this reason I decided to study medicine, and also because I thought the subversive freedoms of studenthood would teach me about life, and medicine was the longest course available at university. My parents, sensing perhaps the unsoundness of my motivation, were less enthusiastic than I'd expected.

'It's a tough profession,' my father said. 'You shouldn't feel any obligation to do it because of us.'

'I always imagined you'd opt for something creative,' suggested my mother generously, perhaps on the basis of the sketches with which I'd illustrated my letters from Israel, 'travel-writing or painting. Once you make a commitment to medicine you'll find it has a way of controlling your life.'

'It hasn't controlled yours,' I pointed out. 'You returned to university to take an arts degree. Once I've qualified I can do the same, or travel as much as I want. Doctors are needed everywhere.'

The first journey that this decision entailed was travelling to Cape Town University, eleven hundred miles away. The train took two days and two nights of rocking transition, like stages in a decompression chamber; from steamy, tropical Durban, through central Natal's grasslands and aloe-studded koppies that had been Boer War battlefields, over the Drakensberg Mountains and the cold Highveld to the diamond town of Kimberley, and then across the Karoo Desert down to gracious Cape Town. Attending lectures in ivy-softened buildings in the mountain's shadow, I missed Durban with a physical ache. I missed Peta more, and my nights in the university residence would be filled with a longing for her that was not dispelled by daylight. When she moved from her parents' Westville home to continue her studies in Johannesburg, a mere thousand miles from me, I began hitch-hiking up for weekends, starting on the highway outside Cape Town at five A.M. on a Thursday morning and – if I was fortunate – reaching Johannesburg twenty-four hours later.

The first six hundred miles of my route lay through the Karoo. Flat-topped ridges and conical mountains would appear on the horizon and take an endless time to draw near, while the tyres fluttered on heat-softened tar and sunlight ricocheted off miles of fractured stone. The only breaks were the lonely desert *dorps* – Leeu-Gamka,

Beaufort West, Richmond, Colesberg – with their main streets wide enough to turn an ox-wagon team and the white steeple of the Dutch Reformed Church sticking up above tin roofs and stunted peach trees. The edge of town would be marked by a truck-stop petrol station and a side-road leading to the coloured township where the workers lived. Sometimes, as I waited for a lift in the middle of emptiness, a family of Nama share-croppers would come clopping by on their donkey cart; the man in a holed felt hat, his woman swaddled in layers of old clothing, while a child or two with yellow skin and high cheekbones sat at the back, their legs swinging. At night they'd sleep by the roadside, their fires flaring in the cold desert wind.

In the course of my migrations I became aware of the social stratifications of these marginal communities. There was an underclass of poor whites, another of coloureds, each jealously guarding their racial status; their superiority to the blacks (a minority in this part of South Africa except in the larger towns like Bloemfontein) and to the Asians, who were forbidden to reside in the Orange Free State province and allowed only seventy-two hours' transit time across its soil. The white and coloured Afrikaners were almost indistinguishable: darkened from the sun, interbred, sharing the same surnames. Hard luck had made them generous, and they'd often stop their battered vehicles to pick me up when I stood stranded at the approach of darkness. Kids would be placed on laps to make room for me inside, or I'd join the huddled figures in the back of a pickup and we'd drive through the night under a brilliant lid of stars while the cold robbed us of all thought. They seemed nomadic – living off roadhouse food, driving with a bottle of Klipdrift brandy between their knees to ease the monotony of their endless journey – and would often leave me in a spot as remote as that in which they'd found me, turning off along dirt roads that led to distant farmsteads.

Peta lived in the Johannesburg YWCA, an institution of rigorous chastity that would not allow me past the front desk. When I was in town, therefore, we had to find other places to be together. In this we were helped by the kindness of students at Johannesburg's Witwatersrand University; inspired by Woodstock and the anti–Vietnam War movement in the US, many embraced a spirit of communalism and hippy generosity. People around campus offered us places to stay in their bohemian houses or smuggled us into unused rooms in the residence halls. Anti-apartheid political rallies in the university's central square would turn into parties that lasted entire weekends. There was a feeling of intellectual fervour, with my medical student contemporaries at the university diversifying into abstruse research in neuro-physiology or astrophysics. At the house of my friend Graeme, a tall, shock-haired drinker and genius, conversations on radical politics ran alongside expositions about memory structure and the properties of quasars.

Leaving Johannesburg was always a sadness, and I would delay my departure until noon on Sunday, when I would kiss Peta goodbye on the side of the highway that ran below the university and stick out my thumb. I'd get rides with men on their way back to jobs on the mines or the railways, in souped-up Impalas and Rancheros with turquoise fur on the dash and Latest Hits on the eight-track stereo. Nursing critical hangovers from another rum-and-Coke weekend, they would barrel through the industrial belt west of Johannesburg to hit the open road where, talking through the night to stay awake, they'd reveal tragedies as profound as any drama.

'That's me,' said a man, opening a twenty-year-old clipping he had taken from his wallet. It showed a picture of a small boy with sticking-out ears, being led into a hall between his parents. The caption described the event as an inquest into the deaths of thirty-two pupils from a farming community, killed on their way to school by an express train when their bus had stalled on an ungated level crossing.

'I wasn't on the bus because I was sick in bed,' said the man. 'I was the only child in the district left alive.' But I could see that he had not survived.

I was seeing more pathology on the road than ever in my studies. Through one long night I travelled with an Afrikaner family in which cousin had married cousin; the line was now ending with their silver-haired children who lay among blankets in the back of the car, blind and deaf and dying of kidney failure from a rare genetic disorder. Another driver, just after sunrise, left the road in a sudden sliding swerve, fishtailing along a dirt track that led into the desert. The car shuddered on the corrugations, trailing dust. The man stopped at a bridge over a gully and reached down beside his leg to produce a bottle of cane-spirit. After offering me a drink, which I declined, he dug an automatic from the glove compartment and, clutching it unsteadily, invited me to step out of the car. I could detect no menace in his tone, only a profound melancholia, so I did as he suggested while hoping that I wouldn't end my life in this empty place. But all he wanted was some company while he drank and shot at the tin cans and bottles in the hollow below. After using up most of his ammunition he offered me the gun, and by pure chance I managed to pop the bottle at which he had aimed his wavering shots.

'My luck is gone,' he said without apparent bitterness, stoppering his bottle. We returned to the highway and the journey west and he put his foot flat, as though trying to run down his shadow that stretched ahead like an inheritance of doom.

Dozing in the back seat of the car of two businessmen, with the prospect of a lift through four hundred desert miles, I was roused by the vehicle braking sharply. The road ahead was strewn with household objects: pots, shoes, a yellow cardigan, a rocking plastic bowl. The trail of debris arced off the tarmac, marked by clothes caught in the scrub, and ended at an overturned pickup truck with wheels in the air and its cab crunched down amongst the boulders. Our driver switched off his ignition. In the silence I could hear a sound like a voice, exhaling a moan of pain with each breath.

'You're a medical student, you said.' He jabbed his chin forward, as though unwilling to lift his hands from the wheel. 'Go and help.'

'Aren't you going to give me a hand?' I asked the men.

'It's your job,' said the driver.

I stepped out of the car, my legs trembling. A terrible fear slowed my footsteps, for I knew that something in my life – an innocence – was ending. Up to now I'd been a spectator, a tourist, reading about death, seeing intimations of its handiwork from a distance. What I was about to find among the scattered clothes would be part of me forever.

The vehicle had been carrying three generations of a family, ten people or more, who now lay smashed across the ground. I had not the first idea what to do, so I went from body to body, trying to count them. Though the children had been flung furthest they seemed least injured; broken arms, gashes, stunned looks on their dust-caked faces through which the blood formed shiny channels. I found a baby with a dislocated knee and brought it to a grand-mother, her grey hair wild, who rested back against a ruptured suitcase, but she held the infant with utter incomprehension as though unaware that she or it were still alive. Three other adults seemed dead. One stuck out from beneath the truck's tailgate which cut across his middle. His mouth was open in an expression of surprise and his face was as purple as wine. A young man and an older one were compacted in the vehicle's cab, their crushed faces visible through the slit of collapsed windscreen. Some yards away a woman lay on the ground, handsome, undisfigured, staring up at me as I approached. She gazed at me with piercing concentra-tion, her lips moving. I leaned close to hear what she was trying to say and became aware of other voices. An ambulance had arrived – someone must have reported the accident in the next town – and its crew was moving, with what appeared to be lackadaisical slow-ness, among the casualties.

'This one's alive,' I shouted to the nearest paramedic, who came over. 'She's trying to say something.'

'*Ag kak,* man,' he said, not unkindly, 'she's long gone,' and I saw now that her eyes were hazed with the opacity of death.

Another ambulance pulled in and, utterly redundant, I went to look for my ride among the cars parked by the roadside. The busi-nessmen had departed, leaving my bag in the dust. One of the rubber-neckers agreed to give me a lift onward and as we drove he spoke about the carnage he'd seen along this stretch of road, de-scribing deaths and injuries with prurient relish. I didn't mention that I was a medical student, for I felt disgraced by my incompe-tence. I couldn't help the outcast and bereft who travelled the high-way, not even with a bit of first aid. I couldn't even diagnose death. It was shame that forced me to apply myself to my studies.

✛

Alongside the physiological mechanisms that sustained life, we needed to understand the corporeal mysteries of the human body.

Every morning we laboured in our group of eight students – teamed four to a body side, one of a dozen similar groups at a dozen dissection tables – dismantling our cadaver layer by layer. He was a sinewy man with tattoos of anchors and palm trees and the names of exotic ports that indicated he'd been a seaman. We tackled the face first, perhaps to remove its capacity for reproach, but the excision of skin from around the eyes gave him a startled expression that only accentuated his humanity. A devout Christian girl in the group trimmed his stubbly beard with her dissecting scissors and passed time, in a dream of contentment, squeezing curls of sebum from the pores around his nose, until all the facial skin was gone.

We revealed the muscles of expression surrounding eyes and mouth, then the supporting ones beneath. The lifting of each layer brought new metamorphoses to the face and its personality: sensitivity, alertness, steely resolve. There were times when it resembled that of the woman by the roadside, others when an incidental asymmetry – our teams worked at different speeds, so that a lip might persist on one half of the mouth while the other already showed only teeth – suggested bizarre caricatures, or explicit evocations of people I knew. Eventually, delivering the eyes from their sockets and slicing under the jaw to draw out the tongue with its root, we were left with bare bone; on my own skull I could feel each ridge and foramen, as though we were identical twins.

Over the course of the anatomy year we got to know our subject well. We viewed his brain, grey-purple and shrunk inside its case, and saw its sections, sliced by the tutor with smooth knife-strokes. His sailor's tattoos we tried to preserve, cutting around them as we flayed the skin from the rest of his body, but eventually they too went into the bags destined for the incinerator. When we turned him over to work on the back a small turd escaped from his anus and the Christian girl cleaned him up briskly. 'Just like looking after my little nephews,' she said. Under our exploring knives the process of dissolution continued, through arms, legs, chest and abdomen. White networks of nerves, picked clean, lay spread like lace on brown muscle.

In our first forensic challenge, we discovered what might have caused his death; a process as complex and enigmatic as what had once made him alive. The bottom of the right lung was stuck down from old inflammation. As we separated it a pink sludge welled up through a hole in the diaphragm.

'Anchovy paste,' murmured our tutor, with the tone of an epicure. Inside the abdomen he snipped through the ligaments of the liver, then dissected it free from the underside of the diaphragm, the jaws of his scissors making little rasping sounds. The liver showed a ragged cavity containing more pink matter. Returning to the right lung, he sliced into the bronchus to show the same sludge. 'This stuff is characteristic of an amoebic liver abscess,' he explained. 'It's said to look just like anchovy paste, which I think you'll agree it does. He probably caught amoebic dysentery on his travels and it wasn't diagnosed. Amoebae get through the gut wall into the liver and form an abscess which grows until it erodes through the diaphragm, then into the lung, so that he's coughing up bits of his liver. His cause of death is recorded simply as pneumonia, so I guess the treating doctors up the hill' – he gestured through the window at the teaching hospital on the mountain's shoulder – 'didn't pick it up.'

The deeper we journeyed in pursuit of death's mysteries, the more He invested our lives. Bits of corpse-fat became pressed between the pages of our anatomy books, making the diagrams translucent. Fragments escaped the dissection room in our shoe-treads to reach the outside world, moving in with us, becoming incorporated in the carpets of our digs and residence rooms. As we pared him down through muscle, nerve and viscera to bone, I too got thinner and thinner. The stench of formalin soaked into my clothes and pickled my fingers. At mealtimes each lifted forkful brought the bouquet of the dissection rooms to my nostrils, and my appetite vanished. When the next academic year began I was not sure that my spirit would survive assault by the hundred thousand facts of bacteriology, pathology and pharmacology. What faltered was my bond with my distant lover.

I betrayed her with a wild girl I met in Cape Town, who wore gypsy scarves and hoop earrings and smoked *Gitanes,* and carried with her an air of cosmopolitan catastrophe. At the age of eighteen, Linda had become pregnant by one of her father's business partners. An abortion was unavailable in South Africa except under circumstances of rigid legality – requiring affidavits from psychiatrists and doctors regarding its medical necessity – so she'd absconded from university without telling her family and fled to Europe, her expenses paid by the guilty man. After terminating her pregnancy in Amsterdam, getting involved in a violent relationship in Paris and starving in a London squat, she'd returned home, repaired the rift with her parents – her father had knocked his business associate cold beside the swimming pool – and been sent to Cape Town University, where she was now incarcerated in the most conservative of the women's residences.

I loved Linda and her history – the wounds of real life, the scars of existence – and she loved me, so we tried to find ways to be together, in spite of the strict curfew at her university residence and the dragon of a lady warden who guarded it. One night I was detected on the roof of a walkway that led to Linda's window; the corgis of the warden set up a torrent of barking as I sprinted along the roof to the place from which I could leap over the perimeter fence, while the harridan paced me below, beating on the gutter with a broomstick. We were caught eventually, *in flagrante*. Linda had signed herself out of the residence, ostensibly to visit relatives but in fact to spend the time with me in my bed, and we were lying one morning in intimate closeness when the door of my room vibrated to a volley of knocks.

'Go away,' I growled. In marched the squat form of the lady warden, who had tracked us down through diligent detective work.

'I know about you,' she declared when she saw my face peering over my lover's breast. 'You're the medical student. Well, you're not going to be one much longer.'

Linda was instructed to return to the residence to pack her things and I received a formal letter to appear before the dean of the university that evening in order to be expelled. Knees quivering, I walked up the steps of his colonial mansion and was shown in to the study where Sir Richard – ex-governor-general of Guiana – waited at his desk. I thought I was done for, but with some scapegrace luck, and because he was a decent man who'd possibly been in a few youthful scrapes himself, I got off with a glass of sherry and an admonition to be more careful.

Tossed thus into each other's arms, Linda and I moved together into blissful cohabitation in a student house below the medical school. But after a year, when I had to go to Durban for some days, she took the opportunity to fuck a handsome friend of mine. Our relationship defunct, she left and moved in with the other man. Linda had kept a set of keys for our house. When I heard them rattle in the lock I'd dive out of the back door and over the fence, to play pinball in a take-away joint down on Main Road until I was sure she'd gone. Each time I returned she'd removed more of the objects and utensils we'd accumulated together, the lineaments of domesticated love. I felt I was going mad with pain, a pain that would worsen if I saw her.

In this state I was doing my 'insanity training', an eight week attachment at Valkenberg Psychiatric Hospital – Devil's Peak stood in blue silhouette through the ward windows – where I'd spend each day talking to the unhinged. Everything they told me seemed entirely plausible. I failed to be surprised by the woman who described how at night the devil inserted people into her rectum: 'grown-ups', she was at pains to insist; not children, in case I thought she was perverted. A paranoid schizophrenic had a button on the palm of his hand that, when triggered, would instantly kill whoever was looking into his eyes. He offered to prove it. I told him I was convinced already, taking care to keep my gaze down on my notes. I believed wholly the farmer who had climbed down from his tractor one day to examine a flower, only for it to turn into a swarm of *miertjie-vliegies* – gnats – and fly away, proving to him that the whole world was made of these tiny creatures, including the crops and the cattle and the doctors and nurses and medical students. My surroundings too seemed to flicker at the edges.

I had moved out of my house and was looking after the flat of an architect friend, down by the rail tracks. He was a kindly man who seemed to understand what I was going through, and when he was away he offered me his place as a refuge. Assuaging my loneliness, I read his books, finding several about the 1964 mercenary war in the

Congo, and saw my thoughtful friend in a new light when I discovered, in the photographs of men and jeeps on rutted jungle roads, the architect's younger face. He'd joined up for the adventure and the diamonds, serving three tours in 5 Commando, the unit led by the legendary soldier-for-hire Major 'Mad Mike' Hoare. I couldn't imagine being a mercenary, but there was a powerful allure in the idea of losing myself in some similarly wild venture. At night I studied the syllabus of drink, sitting up with a bottle of whisky and twenty Texan Plain, watching the fragrant smoke curl away while trying not to think about my erstwhile lover in someone else's bed. Goods trains rattled below the kitchen window and a group of meths-drinkers howled and babbled beneath the bridge over the riverbed. Sometimes a phrase would emerge with perfect clarity.

'Die groot lawaai lê voor ons' – the great tumult is ahead – said a voice. At other times I heard my name. I wondered if this was the symptom of schizophrenia called disintegration of ego boundaries.

After a bad night I would avoid lectures and head up the street to drink coffee at a nearby café. One day I noticed a young woman there, sitting alone, and had taken a seat at the next table when I noticed that she was crying. Silently, her head bowed over her coffee cup, she let the tears stream down to her chin, from where they dropped steadily onto the tablecloth.

'What's wrong?' I asked gently, ready to exchange confidences about the sadness of love.

'My husband's dead,' she said, without looking up. 'He was killed last week near Luanda. The army told us not to say anything.'

'Luanda? In Angola? What was he doing there?'

'Fighting,' she answered. 'There's a war. It's supposed to be secret, but I don't care anymore.'

In 1975, eleven years after Mad Mike's Congo campaign, a new post-colonial conflict was under way, though it took a while for us to learn that our government was directly involved. International news magazines arrived at the news agents' with their contents lists censored by a black felt pen and inside pages cut out. The story wasn't covered in the South African press, which reported only a sudden jump in army road-accident fatalities, but the BBC World

Service began coaching us in the confusing acronyms of a three-sided war. When Portugal had withdrawn from its overseas colonies a few weeks before, Angola's capital and coastal regions had declared for the MPLA (Popular Movement for the Liberation of Angola), the main black liberation force that had been fighting Portuguese occupation for over a decade. But South Africa and the US were determined to prevent a Marxist movement forming independent Angola's new government, and each supported a different faction as their preferred candidate to rule the country.

To the south the MPLA faced the forces of UNITA (National Union for the Total Independence of Angola, slogan: 'Liberty, fraternity, negritude') whose leader Jonas Savimbi – fronted by South African tanks – was fighting fellow black Angolans to free his Ovimbundu people from 'neo-colonial oppression', The FNLA (National Front for the Liberation of Angola) threatened Luanda from the north with the aid of Western mercenaries, recruited through the network of old Congo veterans that had served with Mad Mike Hoare, and paid for with thirty million dollars from the CIA. By early 1976, under MPLA assault, the FNLA's discipline collapsed. Fourteen foreign soldiers, most of them British, were shot for desertion by a British mercenary sergeant, and the scandal of white men killing one another in a black man's war eventually made it into the South African papers. Hoare himself was rumoured to have been wounded and in hiding in Cape Town, being tended by sympathetic doctors. The South African Defence Force was engaged in Angola for the long term. The old law requiring all soldiers who served outside the country's borders to be volunteers had not changed; instead the borders of South Africa had been redefined, for military purposes, to cover all of the continent south of the equator.

✣

Our studies moved on to obstetrics. After lectures and a graphic colour film of a birth that had several students passed out on the floor, we were sent to the Peninsula Maternity Hospital to learn 'baby-catching': how to carry out the fifteen deliveries we were each required to perform as part of our obstetric training. The hospital stood in the wasteland that had once been District Six, the heart of

Cape Town's coloured community until it was 're-zoned' white and the residents deported. Their houses had been bulldozed. All that remained were a grid of streets where stone gateposts opened onto plots of rubble, overgrown with weeds. The only buildings still standing in District Six were the pale green block of the hospital, and a mosque and a church without congregations.

Cape Town's winter had set in, and rain beat on the wards' steel-meshed windows. A veil of cloud streamed constantly down the face of Table Mountain, dissolving always at the same contour, while storm-blown gulls cried in the streets like lost cats. Though its local community had gone, the hospital remained racially classified for coloured use, and patients from Woodstock and Salt River – poor neighbourhoods where coloured and whites yet lived together, the next target of the Apartheid bureaucrats – would be brought to Peninsula Maternity to groan together in the long communal wards until it was time to be moved to the delivery rooms. There, brisk midwives would teach us how to monitor the stages of labour by counting contractions, feeling the belly and checking for the cervix's dilation.

'Kom, mammie, maak asof jy wil aah' – come on, mum, as if you're trying to shit – they would instruct the woman. Then, as the baby began to come, we were positioned between the straining thighs and – between further bellowed orders to the mother – instructed by the midwives in the art of delivery.

The first birth I attended was close to a disaster. The woman, who was having her eighth child, was entirely relaxed about the event but I was terrified, hands shaking, mouth sand-dry behind my surgical mask. The baby's crown had appeared, a cap of wet black curls, and I was looking around to check that the scissors and clamps for the umbilical cord were at hand when something nudged my hip; I glanced down just in time to field the infant – ejected with a single pelvic clench, liked a squeezed orange pip – before it slithered off the table completely. Clumsily I snatched it up, trying to keep a grip on its extraordinarily slippery limbs, while the shock catapulted it straight into full-throated outcry. The mother beamed around her missing front teeth.

'Dankie, Dokter', she said. *'Vertel vir my wat is dokter se naam?'* and when I told her, she announced that her newest son would be

called after me. I hoped good luck would continue to attend its innings.

With half a dozen deliveries behind us, we were sent off in small groups to apply what we'd learned, at township maternity clinics out on the plains called the Cape Flats. The black and coloured townships consisted of rows of matchbox houses along potholed roads, with chain-link fences flying flags of plastic rag. Instead of streetlamps there were eighty-foot pylons like those at football grounds, whose floodlights laid lakes of harsh illumination over the whole precinct. During the day the clinics were staffed by a doctor, providing outpatient services. At night midwives tended the delivery ward. Parked in the compound were a couple of ambulances used to collect women in labour from their homes, or to rush those whose deliveries became complicated to the obstetric unit at the university teaching hospital. After delivering babies, riding the ambulances became our greatest pleasure: hanging on to the stretcher in the back while the siren wailed and we flew around the curves with screaming tyres. When our duties were over, with the patient dropped off at the hospital and the ambulance on its way back to the clinic, we would help ourselves to gulps from the mask of nitrous oxide – laughing gas – and slump helpless and euphoric on the floor. Fortunately its effects were short-lived, so that we were entirely sober when it was time to deal with the next birth.

✛

In mid-1976, shortly after we'd finished our obstetric attachment, the townships became too dangerous to send students for training. We heard the news when we were on vacation, six of us driving a VW bus to Johannesburg the long way round via South West Africa and Botswana: a three-thousand-mile journey that included the Kalahari Desert, the Okavango Swamps and wild, endless bush. The way from Buitepos – Outpost, the last town in South West – to Maun in central Botswana was a track of deep dust, eroding at its edges, becoming overgrown in the centre, over whose ruts and billows we floated on smooth sand-tyres that prevented our vehicle digging in. At night we camped in the middle of real Africa. Lions roared nearby, a deep, reverberating cough that caused the heart to spasm in atavistic fear. Piling more wood on the fire, we listened to the radio reporting flames from the other real Africa; South Africa's townships were burning. Black schoolchildren's protests in Soweto had been met by police gunfire and insurrection had spread to the other townships around Johannesburg before flaring, like a train of gunpowder, all the way to Cape Town.

The vehicle's gearbox locked near Maun – we hoisted it up on a tree, dropped the engine and transmission and fixed the errant selector – and then its alternator burned out at Chobe, so we left it behind and hitched on to Johannesburg. There the atmosphere was electric, Witwatersrand University bristling with anticipation; student activists foresaw the end of Apartheid and they waited for the Revolution to overwhelm the cordon of police surrounding the townships and roll unstoppable down the city's streets. They'd erected barricades at the entrances to the campus and fought pitched battles against the riot squad's tear gas and batons. I found my genius friend Graeme more wild-haired than ever. In an elegant research project he'd successfully taught a task to a tankfull of fish, and with the infusion of radio-labelled amino acids had demonstrated that memory was stored in the fish brain in the form of complex proteins, structured probably in helices like DNA. He believed it could be a breakthrough in understanding the mechanisms of human thinking.

Once back in Cape Town, though, there was no air of revelation. A student militia had been formed at the medical school that patrolled in hard-hats, carrying pick-axe handles and walkie-talkies and their personal firearms. Mobilisation instructions were stuck up on the notice boards requesting volunteers. The night after my return we were sitting in the kitchen of our house around a demijohn of wine, assisting our political theorists in a tipsy analysis of the rising, when the lights went out. At the same instant the air was rent with a deafening roar that set the windows rattling in their frames. We ran, tripping over each other in the lightless hallway, out onto the front veranda.

The streetlamps were off, and even the hospital high on the hill behind the house was dark where its emergency generators had not yet come on. We looked east towards what was normally a sea of light: the white suburbs, the sodium glow of the city's industrial belt, and beyond, the township arc-lamp towers pouring their bleak effulgence over the Cape Flats. Only darkness faced us, and the relentless, bellowing noise that pressed on the eardrums. A few of us shinned up onto the roof. From that vantage it was clear that the whole city was blacked out. Deafened, we shouted questions to each other.

'That's the sound of steam escaping,' yelled someone. 'Maybe they've blown up the power station.'

We stood there, surveying the void where European civilisation had thought itself so solidly established on the continent's tip, feeling the noise soak through us like a torrent of irrevocable change.

The hospital windows were illuminated now by the muted glow of the back-up system. Flashlights could be seen moving jerkily down the flight of steps that led from its parking lot to the top of our street. Their beams twitched across the house-fronts. It was one of the student patrols, and we shouted to them to ask what was going on. At first they could not locate us – the noise confused them – and the lights shrank together. Then, picking us out in their torches where we sat along the ridgeline, they ordered us off our roof.

'Fuck off!' we shouted, throwing them obscene signs, and they continued their march down to Main Road where hesitant car lights passed. Beyond them the roaring darkness stretched unbroken to the sawtooth horizon of the Hottentots Holland Mountains, outlined against the paler eastern sky.

✪

The advent of this shadow brought an unprecedented family gathering. My parents flew down from Durban, bringing with them my brothers and sister. They stayed in a hotel in Seapoint, Cape Town's most cosmopolitan corner, near the Viennese cafés and the Italian Gelateria. The steady evening wind of Cape Town's spring sighed in the palm trees. In the dark-panelled ambience of the Longhorn Steakhouse – I ate voraciously, for the vicissitudes of student life had long since robbed my stomach of fastidiousness – we held our family meeting, and my father announced that he had been offered an orthopaedic post at an American medical school by one of the surgeons he'd worked with in Jerusalem, when they'd treated the wounded together during the 1973 October War.

There were sound reasons for considering this option. It seemed that a time of bloodshed lay ahead, with South Africa engaged in an escalating war against neighbouring countries and within its black townships. The South African Defence Force's casualty lists were growing, and my dad had discovered that his name was still on the Reserve List when they'd offered him the rank of colonel to direct the treatment of military orthopaedic trauma. This was not a conflict that he could support. Instead my family – including my youngest brother and my sister – would leave at the year's end for New York, while I and my other brother, both at university, continued our studies in South Africa. Along with us my parents would leave behind their birthplace, friends and colleagues, professional standing and social regard. To me this tearing up of roots seemed a liberation. I didn't realise yet the importance of knowing where your home is in order to make your path in life. I was setting off on my own adventure.

4

Tropical Diseases

We flew over the sea for a long time. The Mozambique Channel was a dazzle of light, refracted in the lenses of my cracked spectacles. An unready traveller, I had been walking across the apron to board the aircraft in Johannesburg when I panicked that I had lost my passport; looking down sharply to check my pocket, my spectacles had skied off my sweat-slick nose and dived to the concrete. The glass hadn't shattered, but a transverse crack on the right chopped my vision in halves, while a veritable star in the left lens turned everything to fragments. I had no second pair. Squinting at the glinting sea as though through a kaleidoscope, or dropping my chin like a boxer in order to read my book, I cursed my clumsiness and the fearful consequences of choosing to head so far into the unknown.

I knew no-one in the Seychelles. My only contact had been through a letter I'd written to 'The Medical Superintendent, The Government Hospital, Port Victoria, Mahé Island', to ask about working there for my elective – an approved break for medical students to acquire clinical experience before the start of the final year of studies. Most of my classmates had opted for South African rural hospitals or the specialised departments of university teaching hospitals. An orthopaedic colleague of my father's had offered me an attachment within his unit in Hong Kong, but I was in search more of adventure than of knowledge. I'd seen an old guidebook on the Seychelles – ninety-seven or ninety-nine or a hundred and four granite islands and coral atolls, mostly uninhabited – scattered across the Indian Ocean a thousand miles off the coast of Africa. The black-and-white photographs suggested a translucency of sea beneath bowing palms that attracted me powerfully. After many weeks an answer had come from the hospital, a 'flimsy' on which the typewriter had punched out each O and made the stops a pattern of indented Braille. It stated that my arrival was expected and listed the sort of pathology I'd be encountering: tropical illnesses, general medicine and surgery, obstetrics and gynaecology. Venereal diseases, the superintendent had added, were another area ripe for study.

The sea ahead was shadowed by a flotilla of clouds, their tops lit gold by the lowering sun, and I saw that each one capped a ridge-backed island. The aircraft descended slowly over green marching rollers and crossed a line of reef. Granite cliffs rose above the jungle. We banked above a bay studded with islets and the sails of schooners. The town sped towards us, pink and cream and red-rust roofs, as we settled lower over the water. Just when a splash-down seemed inevitable the end of the runway appeared, built out like a causeway, and we dropped onto its solid surface. Blue twilight was settling over the bay, and as our engines sighed into silence the first lights were emerging up the hillside amidst the trees.

The air smelled of my childhood, of salt water and spices and the narcotic scent of some tropical flower. The white concrete airport building with its glass-faceted control tower was the same 1930s design as Durban's old terminal. Within was an air of relaxed confusion, where customs officers handed out arrival forms and poked through luggage at their wooden counters. An official inspected my form and pointed to the empty 'Address in Seychelles' line. I explained to him that I was expecting to be met by someone from the hospital, and did not yet know where I'd be staying.

'Ah,' he said, 'the medical student. Man waitin' for you,' and returned with a slim Englishman in sandals and slacks.

'Giles,' he introduced himself. 'I'm the surgeon. You'll be staying at our place for the first couple of days.' I noticed that he was examining me doubtfully and, realising that my cracked spectacles gave me a rather derelict appearance, hastily explained my accident.

'Takes six weeks to get new lenses from Mombassa,' he said. 'It'll be quicker to call and get another pair sent out to you from South Africa. Come along, then, we'll get home and see if the international operator will pick up,' and he led me out into the warm night.

We drove through the hills above Port Victoria to the Giles's bungalow, where I met his wife, Louisa – explaining my damaged glasses as I shook her hand – and a small daughter in Peter Rabbit pyjamas who nodded at me sleepily before the nanny took her off to bed. I made a call to my mother, busy packing up the family house in Durban, and then Louisa was urging me to change into 'something smarter.' 'There's a do at the British consul's place this evening,' she explained. 'You'll get an idea of how this place operates. Some long trousers and a reasonably un-creased shirt should do it. Oh, and lace-ups, because it's a more formal occasion.'

I mentioned my embarrassment at my cracked spectacles.

'It's a garden party, and people will be drunk,' she said reassuringly. 'I don't suppose anyone will notice.'

A white-shirted policeman waved Giles's car up onto the verge and we ducked through an arch in a great bougainvillea hedge, to be greeted by our host. The consul was a dumpling of a man in a black dinner jacket with a row of miniature medals on his lapel. He shook my hand, his smile already preparing itself for the next arrivals. We walked through to the garden where the buffet was set up. Giles and Louisa were commandeered by friends, while the consul's wife – bronzed and grooved like a kipper – organised me some breadfruit chips and a milky, rum-flavoured cocktail that floated a sprig of greenery and a small crimson flower. I crossed the patio to where the lawn dropped away to a line of dark foliage. Beyond lay the bay, its waters lit by the just-risen moon. Humped islets stood out black. The lights of a steamer at anchor trailed a long reflection. The perfume I'd noted at the airport was stronger here, and I realised that I stood beside a frangipani tree, its fleshy petals scattered around my feet. I breathed in the hot night, dizzy with the risk of becoming lost. I had never felt closer to paradise.

Behind me the party noise was suddenly hushed, and I returned to where Giles and Louisa were standing among the knots of guests clustered about the patio's entrance. They'd formed two loose lines, between which advanced a shortish figure with slicked-back hair and slightly puffy features, in a tuxedo that pulled a little across the midriff. A pair of large men followed at his shoulders, glaring around like bouncers. From among the watchers came some scattered hand-claps. 'That's Jimmy,' murmured Louisa in my ear.

His Excellency Sir James Mancham, president of the Seychelles, was new in office. In the 1950s, after studying law in England, Mancham had returned home to set up the conservative Seychelles Democratic Party with the support of the *Grand Blancs* – the old planter families – in order to maintain the islands as a British colony. Another young lawyer, Albert René, had founded the opposing Seychelles People's United Party, which urged the end of colonial rule and was backed by poorer Creoles and the descendents of slaves from Africa. Over the years Mancham's party had held a slight majority in the colony's Legislative Council, but despite its preference for continued Crown rule, the British government decided eventually to grant the Islands full independence. The handover had occurred in June 1976, a mere five months before I'd arrived. Mancham was nominated president of the new Seychelles Republic with René his prime minister. René stayed at home running the government while Sir James spent much of his time travelling abroad as the dashing head of the world's youngest country. When back home he lived it up in Government House, the former residence of the British governor-general, with all the trappings of a *Grand Blanc* aristocrat.

✛

With the confidence of my new glasses – delivered within a couple of days by an arriving passenger from South Africa – I began to find my way around the hospital. Capped by a tin roof faded rose-pink, the building was a jewel of tropical colonial architecture. An avenue of bottle-brush trees ran up through gardens of hibiscus and ornamental palms to the entrance. The wards were deep verandas that ran the length of its two floors, shielded by roll-down blinds to keep off the sun or the rains. Patients sat on their beds looking out over the bay and playing cards in their pink issue pyjamas. At the centre of the upper floor was the operating theatre, with a raised cupola for cross-ventilation. Ceiling fans inside stirred the air, slow enough for flies to hitch rides on their leisurely blades. Behind the building rose jungle-shadowed cliffs and the pinnacle of Morne

Seychellois, Mahé's highest peak, capped each afternoon in the December clouds of the north-west monsoon.

Under colonial rule relatively few Seychellois had left the islands to go to university, and only a couple had qualified as doctors. Most of the medical staff at the hospital were expatriates from Great Britain. Trained as a surgeon in the British army, Giles was now on contract for a couple of years to the Seychelles government, prior to returning to England and a hospital consultantship. Even with his extensive experience there were surgical situations that he hadn't encountered, and my first role as operating assistant was to read aloud from a volume of surgery and hold up the book while he peered at the illustrations. Routledge, his physician colleague, had spent decades in Africa. He was tall, with a sun-damaged bald spot, and below his white coat his legs moved like those of a wading stork. His field was tropical parasites: hookworm, whipworm, elephantiasis, malaria, schistosoma and river blindness. Some of these were not found in the Seychelles and it was clear that Routledge missed them; sometimes he would reminisce about how the Loa Loa worm travelled across the surface of the eye with a pulsing movement, or the way a boil on a cheek would extrude the wriggling larva of the putsi fly.

Obstetrician/gynaecologist Elsa McGee had rather more exotic pathology than she wanted. Square-jawed, crop-headed for the heat, she was waging a one-person campaign against sexual sloppiness and its consequences. Every outpatient clinic brought new permutations of venereal disease; even genital yaws, called *Framboesia* after the way its lesions stood out from the skin like plump raspberries. The condition was sufficiently uncommon for her to find me on Giles's surgical round and haul me back to her clinic where, parting the thighs of a mortified girl, she pointed out the eruption on a crinkled labium. The beds on her obstetric ward were filled with pregnant teenagers and their pregnant mothers, for liaisons outside marriage were the norm and babies plentiful. The hospital's family planning clinic made little headway against the Islands' Catholic bishop, who railed against contraception on the Seychelles Broadcasting Corporation wavelength. Elsa's richest Scots expletives were reserved, however, for the Evangelical Broadcasting

Agency station whose short-wave transmissions carried ignorance across the Indian Ocean, and the appearance of its white-polyester-shirted personnel at the hospital promised displays of exquisite rudeness.

Mercier was Seychellois, and responsible for anaesthetics. He was a generous chap who'd offered me accommodation in a room in the garden of his bungalow, not far from the hospital. Mercier taught me the essentials of anaesthesia: induction, putting the patient to sleep by injecting a quick-acting barbiturate; and intubation, the vital skill of passing a tube down the trachea of an unconscious, non-breathing patient whose respiration had been stopped with a muscle-paralysing drug. This muscular relaxation was necessary in order to carry out abdominal surgery or major orthopaedic operations, when patients would be connected to a ventilator that would do the breathing for them. Mercier showed me how to set the anaesthetic machine that controlled the mix of gases from the cylinders of oxygen and nitrous oxide in order to maintain unconsciousness in that delicate band between oblivion and death. The supply ship that brought these cylinders was sometimes delayed, so the gases were husbanded for those cases where they were essential, and operations were carried out under local anaesthetic wherever possible.

In the out-patients department one morning I watched Giles examine a man with abdominal distension and a swelling in his groin. Giles prodded his belly and felt the swelling – the man groaned – then tapped the bulge, which resonated like a small drum.

'Hmm. Bombay gas abscess,' he murmured. I nodded knowledgeably, and he turned upon me a critical eye. 'Ever heard of it?'

'Er... no.'

'You shouldn't have. It's an apocryphal condition, a diagnosis attributed to surgeons of the Indian subcontinent. Supposedly, they discover a lump like this in the groin; cut into it, some gas escapes, and the patient dies. Of course, any trained surgeon – and the ones I've met from India are better trained than many – knows that this is not an abscess but a hernia, with a loop of bowel stuck inside it that contains flatus. Simply incising it would release the gas plus intestinal contents, which would run back into the abdomen and cause fatal peritonitis.'

The patient, unperturbed by this exposition, smiled agreeably when Giles said he would take him to the operating theatre to fix the problem.

Relaxed through the administration of a mild sedative, the man watched in the reflector of the overhead surgical light as Giles injected local anaesthetic around the swelling in his groin. The skin opened under the knife to reveal yellow fat, pricked red where vessels were starting to bleed. Giles tied them off. I held the wound open with retractors, while he deepened the incision to expose the layered muscles of the abdominal wall and the defect between their fibres through which the hernia bulged. Its sac of peritoneal membrane looked dull and inflamed. The patient peered raptly into the mirror as Giles injected more anaesthetic around the neck of the bulge and opened the top with his scissors. Cloudy fluid spilled out, then, with assistance from Giles's fingers, the end of a thick red structure like an angry sausage. Its tip was black. The tugging on his vitals had turned the patient quite pale with nausea, but, vomit-bowl at the ready, he was not to be distracted from the parade of astonishing things that were appearing from his insides.

'Aha,' said Giles. The patient and I exchanged glances. Neither of us had ever seen anything like it.

'How many appendectomies have you done?' Giles asked me.

'None,' I admitted.

'Well, this will be your first, and a pretty unusual one, because that's what this hernia has got stuck inside it.'

I was hard-pressed to recognise the appendix: the usual pale tendril of gut was now expanded to this turgid monster, supported by a buttress of inflamed fat like scarlet barley sugar. Giles showed me how to find the blood vessels where they lay within the fat, clamp them with pairs of artery clips and cut between the clips. Under his instruction I tied the vessels so they wouldn't bleed, then crushed the base of the appendix with a heavy clamp and tied around this too, with thick catgut. Cutting off the appendix, I put in a suture in the way that Giles demonstrated, picking up the outer layer of the adjacent bowel wall and gathering it over the appendix stump in a small, neat pucker. The patient gave me a thumbs-up sign, and I blushed behind my mask.

Giles repaired the abdominal muscle defect with a mesh of sutures and closed the skin. With the operation over, he took the appendix out into the sunlit courtyard and cut it open. Lodged inside was a two-pronged fishbone like a devil's horns. This had caused the appendix to become inflamed and swollen so that it was no longer able to slip in and out of the hernia. Instead it had stuck, going black as its blood supply was strangled by the hernia's tight neck. Here was pathology; cause and effect, clearly manifest and simply solved by surgery. One day, I thought, I might become a surgeon, and be able to demonstrate with elegance such examples of nature's perfidy. But that seemed far away, and I hoped to defer responsibility for as long as possible. There was so much else to explore.

✪

Routine hospital work was generally over by three P.M., and I would go back to Mercier's place to pick up my beach things. Tempting though it was to pause for a siesta, I did not linger. Tiffany, Mercier's wife, was usually at home. He had married her while studying in England and brought her back with him. The heat did not agree with her; she'd become indolent, putting on weight. Most mornings she worked as a kindergarten teacher. In the afternoon Tiffany would lounge around the house in a kimono, sipping cocktails and reading sex-novels. She had a stack of these in her bedroom, the stock changing as they circulated among the expatriate wives. Sometimes she would appear at the door of my room as I was changing and thrust a lurid-covered paperback at me.

'Read from page seventy,' she'd say breathily, 'tell me what you think.' Disturbed by the pressure of her breasts behind the insecurely tied wrap, I would grab my swimming things and a book (sometimes the proffered one), throw them into my shoulder bag, and set off up the hillside above Port Victoria.

Here was a network of lanes, bordered by deep storm-drains bridged at intervals by slabs of stone. The tin roofs and dormers of the houses were edged with ornate fretwork and their wooden walls, painted in primary greens and reds, glowed amidst the flowers and fruit-trees. Small shops, shutter frontages folded open, formed caves of bright labels and enamelled signs that advertised Tiger beer and Clipper cigarettes. Higher still the lanes became staircases that climbed amidst tin shacks and great boulders. Eventually they joined the road that led over the neck of Mahé Island to the beaches on the northwest coast.

Beau Vallon Bay was a curve of white sand, backed by casuarinas and coconut palms. Some unostentatious hotels stood among the trees. On the beach was a small palm-thatch bar, and after swimming I would lie on my cloth, reading and drinking ice-cold Tigers while a four-piece combo in hotel uniform performed phonetic renderings of 'Buddy-Rivasoff-Barby-Lone' and other reggae classics. Fifteen miles across the bay great anvils of cumulus would build slowly over Silhouette Island, lightning flickering in their blue depths, while Beau Vallon basked in warm light. I'd swim again and drink another beer and read until the sun sank in a lemon haze at the end of Cap Ternay. Then, staggering slightly, I would commence the two-mile hike up over the switchback road to Port Victoria.

By the time I reached the highest point night would have fallen, swallowing the light from the occasional streetlamps with their pulsating clouds of insects. Frog-calls rang in the roadside ditches like unanswered telephones. Wrapped around by the tropical dark, the last of my afternoon's drunkenness carried me over the crest and down towards the lights of Port Victoria. There would be little point in sobering up, for when I reached Mercier's place he and Tiffany would usually be off for drinks at the house of someone in their expatriate circle and the invitation would include me, for new faces were greatly in demand.

Expatriate social interaction was governed by a hierarchy like that of an army regiment. Their circle – police superintendents, bank managers, Cable and Wireless engineers – were the community's non-commissioned officers, a group to which Mercier had honorary membership by virtue of his teacher wife. Many of the other members had moved with the retreating borders of empire, from Zambia or Uganda or Ceylon. In their bones they abhorred change.

'In South Africa you've got things properly organised,' they told me. 'Can't let the blacks fuck the place up,' and when I expressed my objections to Apartheid I was accused, scoffingly, of 'sounding like one of those damn radicals like René.'

Despite Seychelles' independence they were content – Sir James Mancham was the sort of chap it was possible to do business with, even if they didn't take him very seriously – and the men rather admired the president's playboy image and energetic international promotion of his country as the Islands of Love. His crowning achievement to date had been to get the soft-porn film-makers of *Emmanuelle* to shoot one of their undistinguished sequels in the Seychelles.

The expatriate wives were less amused. They claimed to have heard that Jimmy used the immigration department at the airport as his personal dating service. Allegedly, the customs officers were conscientious at getting their arrival forms filled in by single, attractive female visitors, particularly regarding the address of their holiday accommodation; shortly after they had settled in there would be a knock at the door, a courteous gentleman would present a dozen long-stemmed red roses (flown in daily from Paris), introduce himself as the president's personal private secretary and announce that His Excellency requested the presence of the distinguished guest for dinner at Government House. There they would eat by candle-light on the veranda while serenaded from the garden by the police band. Over the liqueurs, it was said, Sir James might try his luck, and the next morning the woman, flattered or shamed, would reportedly be snapped with the president by the court photographer, her picture to join those of Jimmy's other conquests in his personal gallery.

The story chimed with what I'd witnessed of the president's seigniorial style. He travelled in a cavalcade of vehicles, propped high in the back of an open Rolls-Royce. Police motorcycles, sirens blaring, cleared the way, followed by an escort of big men in sunglasses crammed into the humid interiors of some Renault sedans. On one occasion I'd seen Jimmy standing in his Rolls in the midst of a market-place crowd; he was giving a speech while aides tossed out what appeared to be low-denomination banknotes. The *Grand Blancs* supported him, for he was opening the islands to overseas investors – largely South African developers – who received generous tax breaks to build hotels along the coastline. The South African holiday market was growing. The June 1976 Soweto protests and worldwide TV images of police gunning down black schoolchildren had adversely affected the welcome of South African tourists in Europe. They needed somewhere to go where they could relax, where the hotel staff weren't cheeky, and that was just what the Seychelles was providing.

Not all Seychellois were happy to see their lands sold off and their children placed in service to foreign entrepreneurs, who paid low wages while repatriating every penny of portable profit. A particular aversion to servitude was present among the nation's poorest citizens, the descendents of African slaves, amongst whom foreigners were rather losing their welcome. Walking one evening along the road back from Beau Vallon, I became aware of a group of men sitting on the verge, invisible in the darkness but for the glow of their cigarettes. As I approached they stopped talking.

'Bonsoir,' I called, applying my rudiments of Creole. 'Komman sava?'

Instead of the usual relaxed greeting there came a muttered, incomprehensible phrase.

'Ki?' I asked, 'Monpa konpran.' The words were repeated angrily – an insult – as something whirred by my face so close that I felt the flick of air. The object struck the wall beside me and clattered away, sounding like a heavy bit of steel. I broke into a sprint. Twenty yards further I ducked behind a car in case another missile was flung, and listened for pursuit. Over my pounding heart I heard nothing; most ominously, not even a following burst of laughter.

In Port Victoria, in daylight, it was difficult to believe that anything was amiss. The town was built on a cosy scale of one- and two-story buildings with painted roofs wide-eaved against the sun; men in faded shirts and straw hats sat in rum-shops while the women shopped for fish and cassava in the public market. Outside the old Court House and the president's residence loitered a few policemen in colonial-style uniforms of blue trousers and white shirts and puttees. But there were subtle signs of tension. Men sat in parked cars outside the clapboard building that housed the headquarters of René's Seychelles People's United Party, watching everyone who entered. It was difficult to keep secrets in the Seychelles – the entire population was under fifty thousand – and rumours circulated that those criticising certain government figures risked beatings or even disappearance, perhaps into the sharks that patrolled the roiling undertow of Police Bay.

One night a man was brought to the hospital. He'd been found in one of the storm-water drains that flowed into the harbour and his shirt was soaked with black matter that gave off a vinous stench of rotting copra. His assailants had worked him over with hammers. The man's face resembled a blue melon, the whites of his eyes turned red from ruptured blood-vessels. When we shaved his matted hair the scalp was covered with crescentic contusions like a beaten-metal bowl. Giles drilled into the skull at both temples in an attempt to reduce pressure from bleeding on the brain, but the man's condition did not improve. He lay behind a screen in the ward, breathing stertorously. Sometimes a policeman occupied a tipped-back chair in the corridor; when he was absent a nervous relative, tipped off by sympathetic nurses, would slip in to see the patient. The man snored on, in the cyclical rhythm called Cheyne-Stokes Respiration that indicates severe brain damage. Sometimes it would seem that he had taken his last breath and the silence would hang until the next low, rasping inhalation began. At lunchtime, as I left the hospital gates, I passed the undertaker's man who sat waiting in the strip of shade outside the rum store with a brace of black bottles and, propped against the wall, the coffin and the cross.

✙

At Mercier's place Tiffany was becoming even friendlier, and I was relieved when Giles asked me if I'd like to move back to their relaxed family home. Some evenings I'd eat with them, on others I went out on my own. Avoiding the waterfront taverns favoured by tourists and yachting types, I discovered a bar on the hillside above the town where groups of men – and some rather amateur local prostitutes – sat on an outside terrace under the warm night. American military from the secret satellite-tracking and communications-intercept stations on the mountain drank with tan-suited spooks from the US Embassy. Shifty South African businessmen met Seychellois procurers. There were knots of Frenchmen with crew-cuts and pectoral-hugging T-shirts who might have been Foreign Legionnaires on leave, and the English engineers who ran the transmitters of the evangelical radio station and discussed football all night. Apart from the odd outburst of drunkenness the groups tended to keep their heads close, so that a detectable air of intrigue hung over the place.

I began, on my afternoons off, to extend my explorations. There were not many cars on the roads, but most of them – old Anglias and Morris Minors – had space for a thumb-waving hitcher. I swam in different bays along the coast, floating in translucent water above coral and barred light. Stone-fish, rays and lion-fish lurked there, all capable of deleterious stings, and I kept my feet high. One day on the west side, with the hot roadway cooking through the soles of my sandals, I gave up looking for a lift and ducked into a concrete hotel on its own sliver of beach. Barmen in high-collared tunics carried drinks across the sand. Disregarding the row of wooden loungers, I spread my cloth in the shade of a low-dipping coconut palm, then plunged into the cool water. Returning to my place, I found myself in conversational proximity to a woman who had laid her towel nearby.

Tommy was a journalist, she told me, passing through the Seychelles for a break on her way back to the US after an assignment in Beirut. Despite the pile of *Herald Tribunes* at her elbow she was happy to talk, and with an engaging curiosity – that appeared only partly professional – she soon had me chatting away like an old tropics hand. Flattered, I mentioned my impressions of things festering in the bilges of paradise, and regaled her with the rumours of Jimmy's seduction strategies: the knock on the door, the personal private secretary, the bunch of red roses.

'King James, huh, thinks he can just order people around? What woman would fall for such a greaseball?' She laughed, shaking her head, and called over a waiter for drinks. I was captivated by her worldly style. We arranged to meet for lunch the next day in Port Victoria. At that meal, over sailfish *piment* and sweet-potato chips, I mentioned that I was intending to spend a few days exploring the Inner Islands, and asked hopefully if she'd like to join me. To my delight she agreed, and we sat together over my map, planning the journey.

On the agreed day, pack on my shoulder, I was at her hotel before breakfast to pick her up. Tommy wasn't there but she had left me a note. 'Sorry,' ran her scribble, 'WEIRD thing this morning, just getting out of the shower when knock on my door. Thought it was you, but actually guy from the PRESIDENT's office – King James demanding my company on official tour round islands. Would have said no but I AM a journalist, can't turn down exclusive access!!! Back in few days, see you then. T.'

Wounded by disappointment, I tried to compose a reply of extreme non-irony. 'That's how it goes with the whims of royalty and such,' read the note I left for her. 'Looking forward to inside story.'

Four mornings later, at Giles's house, I was dragged from sleep by the telephone's ring. A half-open eye told me it was not yet light; the call probably meant an emergency at the hospital. Through the wall I heard Giles fumble for the handset.

'Yes?' he demanded. There was a short silence. 'I don't know who you are but you can piss off,' he growled. 'Do you have any idea what time it is?'

The phone was returned to its cradle with a crash. It rang again immediately. This time Giles's answer seemed more modulated. 'Hold on,' I heard him say. There was a knock at the door of my room. Giles stood there, looking puzzled. 'It's for you,' he said.

Trying to think who could be calling me – wondering for an instant if it could be Tommy, but why at this hour, and how would she have found the number? – I wound a cloth round my waist and stepped into their bedroom to pick up the handset from the bedside table.

'Hello, who is this?'

'Is that Jonathan Kaplan?' asked a man's voice.

'Well, yes, but –'

'Hold on,' ordered the voice. I turned to the bed with a shrug. Giles and his wife were sitting up against the headboard, staring at me. I opened my mouth to apologise for the intrusion but suddenly a new voice, high-pitched and authoritarian, was barking in my ear.

'What did you mean by "the whims of royalty"?' it demanded.

'Who is this?' I repeated, non-plussed.

'I am His Excellency, President James Mancham,' the voice declared, 'and you have insulted me. You have insulted the office of the presidency. You have insulted the Seychelles Republic.' His diction had begun to speed up, and now he was fairly shouting. 'You have insulted the people of the Seychelles Republic! You –'

'I, ah, I, ah –' I croaked, but he was tolerating no interruption.

'I will have you imprisoned!' he bellowed. 'I will have you deported! I will make you disappear! No-one will know what happened to you.'

'Your – Your – Your Excellency –'

The man was unappeasable. 'You spy,' he foamed, 'I'll have you shot! No-one will know what happened!' and the connection was cut with an ear-splitting crack. Feeling rather faint, I laid the phone back in its cradle. Louisa and Giles were still staring at me. Louisa spoke first. 'Was that ?'

'I think that was Jimmy.' My voice trembled. 'He says he's going to have me deported and imprisoned. And shot.'

'Don't tell me,' said Giles, 'that this is about one of Jimmy's women.'

I began to explain about Tommy and the island trip and the note. 'A private note,' I stressed, 'a mild joke,' but Giles snorted.

'Nothing's private in this place,' he said, 'no jokes. Sounds like he's really miffed.'

'Let's get dressed and have some tea,' suggested Louisa, 'and Giles can make a couple of calls.' I returned to my room. A few minutes later Giles came in. 'I've just spoken to a friend,' he said, 'senior chap in the police. He says you should pack a small bag, bare necessities, and be ready to travel. He's meeting us at the hospital in half an hour.'

Splashing through the puddles from the night's rain, we swung into the circle at the top of the hospital drive. A man leaned against a blue police Land Rover. He was tall and thin and wore voluminous khaki shorts, and an errant sunbeam lit the orange hair on his knees. Bending like a giraffe, he stuck his long, freckled face into the window of Giles's car.

'McFaddean,' he said, shaking my hand. 'Ah heer you bin messin' aboot wi' one a' Jimmy's gurls.'

I tried to explain about Tommy but he waved my words aside.

'Disnae matter,' he said, 'Important thing is to be away off Mahé for a while, lie low, so you'll no come to his attention. If I wurr you I'd go doon to the schooner jetty and take the first boat that's goin' fookin' anywhere. Aboot two weeks away should do it. When you come back it should all be forgotten aboot.'

Most of the schooners at the dock were at rest with hatches closed, but one showed signs of activity. From a boom, a block-and-tackle was swinging a load of cement sacks onto the deck, and smoke came from the wheelhouse where coffee was being brewed. I asked the captain – in shorts and a black beret, faded to verdigris by the salt – where he was going. 'La Digue,' he said, waving a hand to the north-east.

'Kan?' I asked.

'Tout suite,' said the skipper, and I climbed on board and sat in the forepeak, pulling a fold of canvas over my head against the rain that had already begun to veil the hills over the town. I expected at any moment that a Renault full of sunglasses would come bumping along the dock.

The diesel coughed and water swirled green against our side as we turned away from the dock, the deck throbbing with the engine's beat. Beyond the lighthouse, perched on its shoal, we passed out of the lee of the mountains and into the breeze. Ropes were hauled, sails set on fore- and mainmast. The schooner heeled and began a slow climb and fall over the rollers. We left the rain-cloud's shadow and the sun gleamed all around, lighting the small islands that flanked the channel ahead. The wind freshened, plunging the bowsprit into the troughs. Jib-sails were run up. Flying fish broke from under our stem and fanned out ahead, keeping themselves airborne with a tail-flick on the wave-tops.

Some hours later a blue bulge lifted above the horizon. It grew into a mountain scrawled with jungle, rising above a fringe of coco palms. We passed a pinnacle of fluted rocks surmounted by a cross. The ropes were slacked, sails gathered in, and the schooner wafted silently through water so clear that we appeared to float unsupported above our wavering shadow. The anchor chain roared through the hawse, shedding rust, and the schooner snubbed to a halt some sixty yards from the shore. The beach was overhung by palms, the deep shadow between their trunks giving no hint of what lay behind. Deckhands coiled ropes. "We awaitin' the whaleboat," one of them told me, and pointed to where a grey-painted craft was putting out from a slipway in a haze of smoke. It was a wooden ship's longboat, now converted to diesel, and as it came alongside I saw that its crew wore the uniform of old British Tars – blue bellbottoms and square-neck white tunics – with a gold-on-black ribbon around their straw hats that said 'La Digue Whaleboat'. Passengers and cargo were settled under the vessel's canvas awning and we headed back to the shore.

La Passe, the island's main settlement, consisted of some tree-shaded wooden buildings. Odd houses were spaced along a road of powdered coral and scattered among the trees towards the beach. An ox-cart pulled by a long-horned zebu turned ponderously down towards the landing place. Some islanders, reclining against jute sacks on a trading-store porch, paid me no attention. A hollow feeling in my chest, I sat on the verge with my small possessions and wondered what to do next. I had no experience of exile. On the grass nearby some movement caught my eye: four turtles lay there, turned on their backs to prevent escape while they awaited the butcher's blade. A flipper waved, like a call for help. I jumped to my feet and began to walk along the road through the dappled shadow.

Beneath the trees was a building of stone. A white-uniformed nurse stood on its veranda. Grasping for some sort of sanctuary, I approached and introduced myself as a visiting medical student.

'Dr Godwin is inside the clinic,' said the sister. 'Please to enter.'

Surprised – for I'd been told that the only island besides Mahé with a resident doctor was the second-largest island of Praslin – I was ushered within. The doctor, a tanned, fit-looking man in his sixties, wearing shorts and flip-flops, was berating a contrite patient.

'You silly bugger,' he said, 'that's the third time I'm treating you for clap. No more. *Nicht mehr.*' He made a scissor action with his fingers. 'Next time we'll have to cut it off. *Verstehen zie?*'

The patient, evidently German, nodded. He wore loose, striped trousers and a shapeless T-shirt. Under salt-stiff hair his face was sunburned and peeling, the blue of his eyes so pale as to seem bleached.

Godwin scribbled a prescription and held it out. 'Collect this from the sister. And mind you take all of them, or you'll develop something I can't treat.' The man left, his blue gaze gliding over me with the suggestion of a wink.

'So.' the doctor switched his attention to me. 'Who might you be?'

'Medical student from South Africa,' I explained, 'here on my elective. I wondered –'

'South Africa?' mused Godwin. 'I was in South Africa for a while, during the war. God-awful place called Oribi Military Hospital.'

'What year?' I asked.

''Forty-one, early 'forty-two.' He looked at me. 'What's it to you?'

'I wondered if you knew my father.' I said his name. 'He was there about that time.'

'What?' Godwin stared at me in astonishment. Then he swung round in his chair and picked up the handset of the radio that stood on a table behind him. He grunted some sort of call sign.

'Receiving,' came a woman's voice through hisses and clicks.

'Jo,' he said, 'remember that Kaplan chap at Oribi, orthopaedic surgeon?' There was a silence, and then an affirmative bit of static. 'Well, his son has just walked into the clinic. Bringing him for lunch.'

As soon as the last patient was seen to, Godwin led the way to the beach.

'Jo knew your father quite well,' he said. 'She was a theatre sister at Oribi, assisted him in surgery.'

We piled into the whaleboat where it waited at its berth and chugged away to a two-masted vessel lying at anchor. 'Hospital cutter,' explained Godwin. 'Use it to ferry me to the islands for clinics. It's got a couple of bunks below-decks to bring patients back to the hospital on Praslin.' He indicated an island visible perhaps a dozen miles to the north. 'That's where we live.'

Under engine-power we crossed the strait to Baie Ste Anne. As the boat tied in to the jetty a deckhand brought in the lines he'd trailed behind, and unhooked his catch. He handed one – a substantial copper-red fish with a big mouth – to the doctor.

'Bourgeois, they call it,' said Godwin. '*Bourzwa* in Creole. Good with ginger and garlic. We'll have it for lunch.' The fish was slung into the back of his Land Rover and we set off along a palm-lined track that followed the water's edge.

The meal began with gin and tonics. We ate on the terrace overlooking the bay. After a synopsis of my father's career during and after the war, I explained my contretemps with the president.

'Poodle faker!' snorted Godwin, 'Mountebank! Consider yourself a guest for as long a period of laying-low as you need.'

My room overlooked the beach. It made a long curve around iridescent shallows, in the middle of which was moored the yacht of a Frenchman. He had dropped anchor three years before and never left, and a skein of marine growth now hung below the hull in whose shadow a small ecosystem was flourishing, with schools of tiny silver fish that glinted in the refracted sunlight. Each day I would accompany Godwin to ward-rounds and outpatients at the small hospital on Praslin, and twice a week we'd be taken by the cutter to the clinic on La Digue. Despite my lack of clinical experience, Godwin discussed each case with me and made me feel included in the decisions about patient care. I was even able to help in practical ways; one night I sat up stitching lots of little, deep cuts on the cheeks of a drunk Pralinois who had been slapped vigorously about the face by his wife with an unscaled fish.

In the evenings we sat on the terrace while the moon rose and the sea reflected the stern-flares of boats fishing along the reef, and we talked. The Godwins' decision to retire to the Seychelles was the latest of a series of adventurous choices. They'd lived in Oman during a period of unrest, when the British community had been besieged in the Residency compound by hostile mobs. The men had armed themselves with odd weapons; they'd intended, said Jo with a laugh, to reserve their last shots for the womenfolk to avoid 'dishonour'. Godwin also talked about working as a police surgeon after the war in the British Protectorate of Basutoland, during an outbreak of bizarre killings. Corpses turned up, mutilated, victims of 'medicine' or '*muti*' murders in which body parts had been removed to make magical concoctions that were believed to confer invulnerability or spiritual power. He described riding up into the mountains with an escort of Basutoland Mounted Police to carry out autopsies, the body laid on a rubber sheet beside a stream while he recorded the mutilations – fingers, tongue and testicles removed – and dissected internal organs, rinsing them in the icy water to determine the cause of death. Godwin's descriptions, couched in the forensic phrases of a pathology report, were nonetheless gruesome enough for me to put aside my drink, for it seemed suddenly that a mortuary stench lurked under the faint odour of tropical rot that rose from the foliage on the slope below us. Swallowing my nausea, I made some anodyne comment about the incongruity of hearing such stories in this exquisite place.

'It's close to perfection,' agreed Jo, 'though even here you'll find some pretty weird things.'

Jo was a painter and her palm-thatch studio was full of studies of the Vallée de Mai in Praslin's interior, and the giant coco-de-mer palms that grew only there in the whole world. Mystical powers were attributed to the place. The military adventurer General 'Chinese' Gordon, commanding British forces on the island of Mauritius, had visited Praslin in 1882 and declared – on the basis of Kabbalistic decodings of the Book of Genesis – that the coco-de-mer had been the Tree of Knowledge and the Vallée de Mai the original Garden of Eden. A year later the English botanical artist Marianne North arrived in Praslin after having travelled through Brazil, the Caribbean and Borneo, and pronounced it 'the most perfect situation I ever was in'. She painted the coco-de-mer's twenty-foot fan-shaped leaves, the double nut of the female tree shaped precisely like a woman's hips and the purple-flowered phallus on the male palm. But soon she began hearing voices and was invalided home to England's mild light, where her paintings were quarantined in a special gallery at Kew's Royal Botanical Gardens. Jo told me that the islanders believed the cocos-de-mer upped roots at full moon and danced on the beach in a copulating frenzy. Despite the British colonial authorities having formally banned sorcery and charm-making in 1958, voodoo seers known as *bonhommes du bois* were still feared for their ability to make the jungle spirits do their bidding, and on the island of La Digue practitioners of the secret black magic called *grigri* held ceremonies deep in the back-woods; Jo herself had heard the drums.

I thought it would be interesting to stay a couple of days on La Digue. After Godwin and I had finished a clinic on the island, he took me to the house of a local woman near La Passe who would rent me a room. I dined that night in a rum-shop, on grilled fish and plantain, while flying beetles smacked against the glass of the primus lamp and dropped, stunned, onto the table. Raucous parrots had me up at dawn. I bought bananas and mangoes in the market and wandered southward through the serried palms of a copra estate until the sand road turned into a path that continued over a low headland. Beyond, it skirted a succession of deserted silver beaches, where sunlight set the shallows flaming green. By afternoon great bruised clouds had gathered out to sea and I lay on the sand watching lightning strike the waves and rain swallow the headlands one by one. Sheltering in a cave of limestone boulders, I read and ate fruit while the deluge thundered on the palm leaves.

The rain had moved on and I was strolling back through La Passe when someone hailed me. I looked around to see the German who'd been Godwin's patient, dangling some fish on a loop of palm-fibre. Showing me the location of his shack on the beach, he invited me to eat with him that evening. I returned at sunset carrying bottled beer, which we opened while the day's last light tipped the jungle-covered crest behind us. My host set a match to stacked driftwood that flared yellow and sea-green in the growing darkness and we had another beer while the flames subsided to pulsing embers. He anointed the fish with a mash of chillies and ginger and cooked them quickly, a few minutes aside; we ate them with our fingers, listening to the boom of surf along the reef that made a faint phosphorescence in the night. The German went up to his shack and returned with a bottle stoppered with a stick.

'*Calou*,' he said. 'Palm whisky. Wery good.'

I offered him a cigarette, which he used as mix to roll a giant joint. Lighting it with a twig from the fire, he settled himself back on the sand. The toddy fizzed on my tongue.

'Do you believe about *grigri*?' he asked.

'I don't know,' I answered. 'And you?'

'*Ja, ja,* I believe. They are there.' I saw the coal of his joint make an arc as he indicated the jungled slopes that rose black against the stars. 'They put things in the cemetery, you can see: small *puppen,* piece of mirror, bone, feather. They visit there at night. One time I am sleeping on Anse Cocos in east of the island. There is a village there all empty, the houses fallen. I am sleeping on the beach and I hear the drums – big drums, deep, and fast one: *k-tak-k-tak-k-tak.* I go to watch on the side, where there are others watching. In the middle there is a fire and the men were dancing.' The German got to his feet. 'They dance like this.' He rocked and stamped, his striped trousers flashing in the fire-light. 'One man dance and he is leaning back like he must fall but he doesn't fall. In his hand there is a machete making flick, flick. His shoulders are on the sand but his legs still stamping, like an insect; he is near me and I can see that his eyes are white, just white. The *grigri* man threw water on him. It makes steam as it touch him, like he was hot iron. I saw this myself.'

The German took a long drink from the toddy bottle. 'The people say he is *dondosya,* a zombie.' He concentrated on rolling another joint. 'People here say that bad things are happening in Mahé,' he said, 'that *dondosya* working for the president. That is why I stay here on La Digue. The girls are wery friendly, and the doctor makes always complaints but he gives me good antibiotics.'

The next morning, on my way to join Godwin in the clinic, I passed the old cemetery. Crossing a bridge over a weed-choked stream, I walked through dew-wet grass to where the oldest graves – stepped blocks of coral, tumbled crosses – were disappearing into the fringes of the jungle. One was anointed with feathers from a chicken's breast and some tarry substance that gave off a penetrating smell of putrefaction. Deeper under the trees, beside a lichen-blackened crypt tipped by subsidence like a sinking boat, I found a tobacco tin containing bird-bones and shells and tiny parcels of bound bark. A sudden sound, like a deathbed groan, made me jump. The sound was repeated and through the trees I saw a man labouring up the road on a rusty bicycle, its un-oiled wheels protesting. I reached the clinic, and the everyday problems of coughs and coral cuts, with a measurable relief.

◉

After a fortnight, as the police inspector had advised, I returned to Mahé. An envelope had been left for me at the hospital by Tommy, a farewell note asking why I had vanished and giving an address in Washington, DC. No other correspondence reached me for the rest of the time I was in the Seychelles; the letters I'd been receiving from my friends and family were now all intercepted by the authorities. I felt bad about bringing problems for Giles and Louisa and thought it best not to move back into their place, so I found a small guesthouse high above Port Victoria off Crève Coeur

Break-Heart – Road. Each morning I would walk down to the main avenue and jump aboard one of the open trucks with bench seats that served as buses. Through the day I immersed myself in hospital learning. Outside work, my time was taken up by my burgeoning social life.

The guesthouse was an eccentric place, owned by a retired Cornish sea captain and run by his Seychellois missus. Plank-walled rooms in pink and green opened off a central walkway. The shower was a wooden cubicle set against the flank of a giant boulder. Its top, reached by a staircase, was edged by a low wall that formed a belvedere for drinking sunset beers bought from Madame's fridge. The rooms were rentable by the hour or by the night, and each morning before I went to the hospital I would leave my bag in the parlour so that my room could be hired out for daytime activities. Madame employed a pair of girls who cleaned the place, made the beds and went to the market for the captain's dinner. One of them, Monique, became a friend of mine, and when she found out I was working at the hospital she began to consult me on medical issues involving her friends. All their problems seemed to be pelvic – concerns about being unexpectedly pregnant (not apparently a very serious problem) or infertile (extremely serious) or perhaps having caught a venereal disease – and being good Catholics they preferred not to be seen queuing outside the hospital's gynaecology clinic, for it also provided the family planning service and a person's purpose in being there could thus be misinterpreted.

Initially our consultations were verbal and theoretical. But one weekend, when I was reading in my room – rain, pounding on the tin roof, had made it worth paying Madame for the space through the day – the door opened to reveal Monique with a pretty friend in tow.

'This is Camille,' she said. 'She has been trying *longtemps* to get baby.' I started to explain about infertility testing but Camille shook her brown curls; she had heard from Monique that I was a *médicin Anglais, tres sympathetique,* and she wanted me to examine her. Monique had closed the door and disappeared, leaving me with a suddenly naked girl on my bed. I tried to preserve decorum by covering her with the bedspread and doing something innocuous with her pulse. She pushed the coverings below her pubis. I plucked them back.

'Look,' I said, 'you really ought to see a specialist.'

Camille took my hand and pressed it between her thighs. At the same time she turned her face to the wall as though preparing herself to endure the experience in a spirit of martyrdom. I tried to conduct a formal gynaecological examination, while she gasped and thrashed her hair about. Nothing, so far as I could tell, appeared out of place. I covered her again and announced the good news. Camille remained on the bed, unspeaking. I suggested that she get dressed. She shook her head, and I had to get Monique to escort her from my impromptu consulting room. I felt pretty stupid.

The next time I met Camille she was on the arm of a Scandinavian traveller; I assumed his treatment for her problem of being unable to get babies was more effective than mine. She'd brought him to a nearby church hall where Monique had started taking me in the evenings to go dancing. Unlike the bands at the beachside resorts, who tried to sound Electric with their mouths or did touchingly approximate renderings of overseas hits, these musicians played local music. Monique taught me the *sega* shuffle and the more explicit hip-thrusts of the *moutia*. She introduced me to her friends, women with the striking diversity of traits that make up the Seychellois: dark, coffee-coloured, fair, even Chinese. I danced with them and bought them soft-drinks, for alcohol was not served on church property. The girls would whisper together in Creole, then one would announce that she was coming back to the Captain's with me and drag me away.

In my bed they always insisted on having the lights off. They had smooth, firm bodies like India-rubber and an unaffected, earthy counterthrust when they fucked. In the mornings the girls would wake at dawn to avoid Madame, pull on their clothes and be gone, to dash home for a wash and change before heading to work or school. A couple of nights later I'd meet them again at the dance hall, laughing as they urged a friend to go with the *docteur blanc*; Monique told me that my skin colour, and assumptions about my braininess – based on the fact that I wore spectacles, the only time these have proved a social asset – made me a good proposition for fathering a child. Even Monique tried it one morning, slithering as though pre-soaped into the shower where I stood under the tepid stream before going to work, and rubbing herself against me with much more energy than the hour warranted.

✪

I could have stayed in the Seychelles forever. At the hospital my clinical understanding was growing every day. One afternoon a man was brought in by his family from a distant island, carried up in the back of a truck from the schooner jetty. About a week before, he'd suffered a coral cut, which had appeared to be healing. Now the man lay on a metal gurney in the outpatients department, staring upward, apparently unaware of his surroundings. Dr Routledge touched his arm. The corners of the patient's mouth pulled into a peculiar down-turned grimace. His eyes bulged, and a violent convulsion arched the man's back off the trolley so that only his head and his heels pressed, jerking, against the metal top. From his throat came a clacking sound as though some ratchet were being wound to unbearable tightness inside him.

'Tetanus,' said Routledge. 'He can't breathe. Get the anaesthetist.'

The man's family – a woman and a boy of perhaps eight – watched fearfully while Mercier injected a muscle-paralysing drug to prevent further spasms and passed a tube down the patient's trachea. A rubber air-bag was connected, which Mercier squeezed rhythmically. The chest rose and fell.

The situation was stark. The only ventilator in the hospital was that on the anaesthetic machine, and the bottled oxygen that it required had to be conserved for surgery. If the patient was to be kept alive until the crisis was past, he'd have to be ventilated by hand, by the ward-staff, taking three-hour shifts. My turn came in the small hours of the night. I sat down by the bedside and took the air-bag from the nurse, hoping desperately that she would decide to stay and oversee me at work, but her footsteps faded down the corridor and I was alone with the responsibility of this man's life. A small lamp on the bedside table lit his face and the tears that glistened beneath his eyelids.

His wife, exhausted, slept on a cot against the wall. The child was awake, and watched me from the other side of the bed, only his eyes visible above the mattress edge. I squeezed the bag steadily. When cramp locked my fingers I alternated hands. For an hour I stood to hold back sleep, shifting my weight from leg to leg. No sound came from the wards. Outside, I could hear the leathery flap of the fruit-bats. A breeze through the shutters revived me. I sat again, kept squeezing, listening to the soporific sighing of the air-flow. I counted breaths.

A high cry shocked me into wakefulness. I blinked, disorientated; had the man shouted, despite his paralysis? Then I saw the child staring at me, his eyes wide with terror: between us lay his father, whom I had almost let die through my faltering fingers. For an instant they refused to work, fixed in spasm, while my heart hammered against my ribs. I wanted to jump up, to flee from this relentless duty. Instead I unlocked my hands and squeezed the bag, again and again. Infinitesimally slowly, breath by breath, another hour passed. Between the shutters a glow lay along the horizon. The child watched me, unblinking.

There were sounds from outside and Mercier stuck his head around the door. I felt like shouting with relief, but only a croak came from my throat. Hoarsely, I told the anaesthetist how difficult it was becoming to compress the bag, because my hands were so tired. Mercier examined the man, assessing the tone in his arm muscles.

'He's resisting the ventilation,' he said, taking up a syringe. 'The relaxant must be starting to wear off. I'll reverse the drug and we'll see what's happening.'

The patient gagged around the tube as Mercier withdrew it. He opened his eyes. There were no convulsions. His wife fell sobbing onto the bed.

'He'll be okay,' Mercier said to me. 'Go and get some sleep.'

As I left I was aware of the boy still staring at me. He had saved his father's life.

✛

The monsoon had settled in. Each afternoon saw the build-up of vaulting clouds and a tension in the air that discharged itself in pounding rain. It could be heard striding down the hillside; drumming on tin roofs, rebounding off the street and roaring in the storm-ditches. I would sit on the step eating mangoes, cooled by the spray, washing my hands under the water that spouted from the down-pipe. The evenings were clear and I'd lounge on the guesthouse balcony atop the boulder, drinking beer and talking to the other residents, before going off to immerse myself in the night's delights. I knew that my time here was ending, for soon the academic year would commence at Cape Town University, but the lure of this tropical life drew me like a precipice: forgetfulness, absolution from the leaden, penitential demands of career and ambition. Sealing away the fantasy, I went one morning to the travel agent's office near the war memorial and booked my flight. I began making my farewells.

On my last day at the hospital I walked into the gynaecology clinic to say goodbye to Elsa McGee, whose wit and candour had so entertained me; I was sorry that I hadn't spent more time in her department. She wasn't there, so I asked the pair of senior nurses who ran the clinic to convey to Elsa my good wishes. As we were talking I was greeted by a girl who sat in the outpatient queue.

'That one, she regular attender here,' said Big Matron. 'How you do know her?'

'From the dance hall.'

'Have you sleep with her?' she demanded.

Taking my hesitation for shame – in fact I was just, for the instant, unsure – Matron advanced, driving me with her bulk back into the treatment room.

'You sportsmen all the same,' she said, cracking an ampoule of penicillin. 'Drop you pants.'

'Shouldn't I have a blood test?' I protested. 'I mean, I don't have any symptoms.'

'If you know that girl, we got diagnosis already,' she said, chuckling grimly, and she and her colleague took their revenge on the fecklessness of men by jabbing an agonising dose of antibiotic into my left gluteus and a smaller but even more excruciating one into my right deltoid. Hobbling, I made my exit.

The afternoon squall drenched us as we made for the boarding steps of the Air India Boeing. It surged along the runway and hauled itself into the heavy air. A shaft of sunlight, glancing over the mountain's shoulder, set aglow the variegated greens of the reefs in the bay below. I craned my neck to keep the islands in sight as long as I could, but within minutes nothing was visible ahead or astern but an endless vista of sea. Sitting awkwardly, trying to guard both the afflicted half of my rump and my tender shoulder against pressure from the seat, I reflected that there were more apposite ways to take one's leave of Nirvana. In my bloodstream the antibiotics warred against shadowy pathogens: medical science versus sensual sin.

My flight involved a stop-over on the island of Mauritius, where I wandered through the public gardens of its capital, Port Louis. Tufted aerial roots hung from the trees. On a pedestal stood a statue of Brown-Sequard, the nineteenth century French-Mauritian neuro-anatomist who had elucidated the arrangement of different nerve fibres in the spinal cord. I tried to remember the features of the syndrome that bore his name: an injury to one side of the cord produces loss of sensation on the side below the damage, and of vibration and temperature sensitivity on the other, or was it muscle power on one side and spatial awareness on the other? I wondered if he'd ever researched the existence of zombies. Slightly delirious, I allowed myself to be carried back to Cape Town Medical School.

5

Breathing Difficulties

My classmates seemed to have spent their elective periods hard at work improving their knowledge rather than falling foul of presidents, through I did have the personal gratification, less than five months after I'd returned to university, of hearing that James Mancham's tenure as president of the Seychelles had come to an abrupt end. On 5 June 1977, twenty-five days short of his first year in office, he was away attending a grand dinner at a Commonwealth Heads of State Conference in London when a quick coup deposed him from power. Twenty Tanzanian soldiers led by René took over the studios of Radio Seychelles, the government buildings and police headquarters. One policeman died, two were wounded and a new social order was proclaimed. Jimmy's picture collection at Government House was reportedly binned, with the hero of all those conquests now in unhappy exile. I felt a sharp regret at having missed the event; Godwin would, I was sure, have a great story to tell.

Even as the rest of the class plunged into intensive revision I read my books distractedly, finding diversion in overhauling the engine of my truck and sleeping late in my girlfriend's arms. Debra lived with her two sisters in a cabin on stilts, built among the tall pines at Constantia Nek where the road crossed the mountains forming the spine of the Cape Peninsula. The women lived in a state of bohemian rigour. During the day they attended lectures at the university. In the evenings they waited tables at the rustic restaurant for which their cabin constituted staff quarters, and feasted afterwards on bottles of accumulated wine-leavings. There was always a platter of bits of steak and chicken that had been collected by the girls as dog-scraps. With these they sometimes fed other indigent students and there was often a bloke or two hanging about, enjoying the sisters' hospitality.

The cabin contained two beds. If I gave up late on my halfhearted studies and drove up the mountain to Constantia I sometimes found Debra's bed being shared by her formidable sister Jacqui, who would object to my arrival under the covers. Jacqui was taller than me and stronger, and sometimes a wrestling match ensued, with one sister hanging on to me, the other trying to hurl me out of bed. Jacqui usually surrendered after dealing me a whack on the ear that made my head ring, then stepping magnificently over to the sofa, talking the duvet with her. In the small hours of the night the trees groaned and flexed in the wind that came up between the cabin's floorboards to balloon the rugs. Daylight brought the forest alive with birds, and the creep of sunlight up the valley from the east. Of all the time I spent in Cape Town, those days – my awareness heightened by the looming fear of the final examinations – seemed the most intense; a final refuge of youth, a flight from reality, trying to refuse the burden of growing up. In July, during the mid-year break that most of my classmates saw as an opportunity for ever more heightened study, I went to visit Debra and Jacqui where they were taking their vacation in Lesotho.

This mountainous, inward-looking country had fascinated me even before I'd heard Godwin's forensic stories of pre-independence Basutoland. The capital, Maseru, was a frontier town. Colonial-era buildings of rough sandstone lined the main street, their tin roofs glinting in the clear mountain light. Men in conical grass hats, shoulders swathed in blankets, clopped past on stocky ponies. While I'd been at school my father had begun spending periods at Maseru's Queen Elizabeth II hospital as a volunteer orthopaedic surgeon, and we sometimes joined him for a family weekend. His acquaintance with a police superintendent led my brother to be invited on week-long horseback patrols into remote parts of the kingdom with the Lesotho Mounted Police, with their colonial-pattern slouch hats and bolt-action rifles from the British era. An introduction to the health minister had resulted in my working as a young medical student with the country's Flying Doctor Service. If I had been any good at the game I might even have got to play tennis with young

King Moshweshwe the Second, who had returned from Oxford to find that his ceremonial role as head of state left him plenty of time to perfect his service on the specially built courts in the palace grounds.

The police superintendent had shown me round a warehouse stacked with guns, confiscated in recent police searches. Most were of interest only to collectors. There were flintlock muskets, obtained by the first King Moshweshwe to defend his stronghold against the raids of Boer *voortrekkers* in the 1830s, and later Enfield muzzle-loaders taken as pay by Basotho workers on the Kimberley diamond fields in order to resist land-grabs by the Boer Republic of the Orange Free State. Snider carbines and Martini-Henrys dated from the so-called Gun War, when the authorities of Britain's Cape Colony decided to disarm the Basotho by force, only to lose more weapons when a British cavalry column was overwhelmed at a high pass south of Maseru that is still called Lancer's Gap. General 'Chinese' Gordon, posted from Mauritius in 1881 to end the war, spent four months in Basutoland and concluded that the fault lay entirely with the Cape administration. 'It is impossible to act against natives who I believe are being treated unjustly by defective government,' he wrote in his letter of resignation.

South Africa was mixed up in the twisty political conflict now under way. Pre-independence elections in 1965 had brought a narrow victory for the conservative Basutoland National Party, which won with strong support from the Catholic Church, and a year later the BNP leader Chief Leabua Jonathan became Lesotho's first prime minister. The South African government was delighted when Jonathan refused to surrender power after his party lost the 1970 elections to the progressive, pro-ANC Basutoland Congress Party (BCP). Instead he arrested their supporters and declared a state of emergency, enforced by the automatic weapons of the paramilitary Police Mobile Unit, which roared around in armoured Land Rovers. BCP elements had attempted a coup in January 1974, the sounds of gunfire coming across the drift on the Caledon River that formed the frontier between the two countries to where we were staying in a family motel on the other side. The next day we'd driven over the border bridge into Maseru. The avenue that fronted the king's palace was sharp with eucalyptus from bullet-ripped branches that littered the roadway. The Lesotho Mounted Police guardhouse at the tennis court gates had lost chunks of brickwork to automatic fire; quite a lot of it appeared to have come from the PMU station down the road, which sported some pockmarks in return. The British Council offices had been hit generally by both sides.

Since that time Chief Jonathan had begun developing links with the ANC, while fighting a low-grade insurgency in the mountains and townships against BCP guerrillas now backed by South Africa. None of this deterred the fun-seekers. White South Africans from the stuffy towns of the Free State and government bureaucrats from Pretoria and Bloemfontein flocked to Maseru for the weekends. The place was a playground, out of reach of Calvinist moralisers. One-stop decadence was available at Maseru's Southern Sun Hotel: gambling at the casinos and porn in the cinema. In the skin-searing cold of Maseru's winter nights, black prostitutes in tiny dresses clustered outside the bars, vying for the banknotes of stout Afrikaners. Most of Maseru's expatriate population lived in a strange sub-world. Debra and Jacqui were staying with an Anglican priest resident in the country for twenty years, a refined bachelor whose house boarded a succession of handsome black boys that attended the town's equivalent of an English public school. Dressed in uniform of dark blazers and grey flannels, they waited table and poured the cocktails and shivered in the unheated pantry between courses. I understood that they were warmed up before bed with a nightly caning by their guardian in anticipation of any misdemeanour.

We drove north out of Maseru and through the town of Teyateyaneng, where 'Chinese' Gordon had his headquarters during the Gun War. The market was a burned-out ruin following a PMU operation. Following Jacqui's directions – she knew the country well, having worked there as a teacher – we took a dirt road that wound up into the mountains. On the edge of a valley where cattle grazed on pale winter grass, we stopped for a picnic. The cooker and coffeepot were carried up the hillside and sandwiches sliced from trading-store bread. While the coffee brewed, I took a photograph of Jacqui where she stood with the sun behind her, back-lighting her hair and the collar of her sheepskin coat. Printing the picture later, I found that the black-and-white film had given a radiant edge to the grass-tops and to the blanket-wrapped herd-boys and their lean dogs that stood along the slope below, but it was Jacqui's face that was most striking: surrounded by a numinous halo, her features caught in an instant of ethereal loveliness.

✛

Late – almost too late – I returned to Cape Town and immersed myself in the churning race towards Finals. With a fear-honed clarity of thinking that had eluded me through most of my studies, I carved out from the great swamp of accumulated academic information a minimalist syllabus, which I committed myself to understanding. I was helped by friends who had begun this process of concentration months before, and by cigarettes and coffee and carefully apportioned rest. The written papers were manageable, for there was a sufficient choice of questions for me to be able to pass. I contemplated with dry-mouthed terror the approaching oral and clinical examinations, where I anticipated the ruthless exposure of my ignorance. The thought robbed me of sleep and by the time the clinicals arrived I was so exhausted that on one occasion, after completing my assessment of the patient, I sat in a chair at the bedside while waiting for the examiners to appear, and fell asleep.

Luck and kind strangers took pity on me. The woman who was my major case for the gynaecology clinical whispered to me what was wrong with her, and even that there was a dispute between our professor and the visiting examiner regarding the state of her left ovary. All I had to do was to present my findings with a degree of honest-seeming doubt – that ovary, I thought, might be enlarged – for a small smile of superiority to hover on my professor's face as his boy demonstrated to the visiting academic the standard of clinical acumen pertaining at Cape Town University. My medical case was a playful lad with some sort of heart problem. While I struggled through his history, in Afrikaans, he dismantled my stethoscope and palmed the diaphragm; during the subsequent examination I couldn't understand why I could hear no heart sounds until I noticed the translucent plastic disc glinting on his forehead, where he'd stuck it with saliva. Shouting with laughter, he capered round the bed until suddenly overcome with breathlessness. His lips blue from lack of oxygen, he squatted on his haunches, and within twenty seconds his breathing had eased and the pallor around his mouth returned to a healthy pink. At once I remembered the name of the rare condition associated with this response. Fallot's Tetralogy is a combination of four separate congenital heart abnormalities; squatting squeezes blood from the lower body back to the heart at sufficient pressure to push it through a defect in the wall that usually divides the left and right sides of the heart, allowing it to reach the lungs where it is re-oxygenated. Clapping the bits of my stethoscope together, I had just enough time to note the musical array of murmurs produced by the heart's abnormal circulation before the examiners returned and asked me to present my findings.

But in the oral sections of the examinations, being questioned by hard-nosed professors, the void I knew to exist in my academic knowledge choked me with fear and I stumbled and croaked my way through medical and obstetric answers while sweat splashed down my flanks. The glass jar I was given in my surgery oral contained a wrinkled, gnarly structure like an ancient tuber; inverting the specimen launched a snowstorm of sediment. I replaced it on the table and watched the cloud refuse to settle. The examiner watched it too, an eyebrow cocked, waiting for me to speak. I had never expected to get this far through medical school; I considered that I'd had a damn good time, all things considered, and now it was over. There was silence but for the sound of the professor's breath whistling in his nose.

Before the examination results were released I had left Cape Town with my friends David and Liz to drive with them up to Johannesburg. David was expecting to go north across the Rhodesian border to a house officer (intern) post at a hospital in Bulawayo, Liz to meet up with her lover Neil, who had graduated the year before and was now working as a doctor for a trade union representing black workers in the gold mines around Johannesburg. I'd known Neil well, for he'd lived in the student house into which I had moved during the early years of my medical studies. He had been one of the political activists whose conviction had impressed me during long discussions around the kitchen table, though I'd never acquired his taste for lentils. En route to Johannesburg we phoned a classmate back in Cape Town, who told us our examination results.

I'd known that Liz and David would get through – they'd always shown the sort of application and gravitas that the career required – and I'd grown up with clear enough role models in the form of my parents and their colleagues to know how far short I fell of these standards. All through my time at university I had awaited the exposure of my unsuitability, through some lapse or malfeasance that would excuse me further studies on the grounds of an insufficiency of medical fibre. Suddenly, without adequate psychological preparation, I was a doctor. David offered me some reassurance.

'The trick is to listen a lot, look sympathetic and nod slowly,' he advised. 'Remember, Hippocrates said the art of medicine lies in amusing the patient while nature takes its course.'

Doctor David and I drove Doctor Liz to Neil's place, an old farmhouse off the Pretoria road. A tin-vaned windmill clanked outside the kitchen door, pumping borehole water into an irrigation tank. From it Neil filled the kettle and made us tea. It was clear that his life was as abstemious as ever. He offered to put us up on the farm for a couple of days if we wished, but we could see that he and Liz were dying to dive into bed, and said farewell.

Pre-finals, there had been a fever of competition among ambitious fellow-students for house officer posts at the Cape Town University teaching hospital of Groote Schuur. My uncertainty about my prospects had made my own enquiries more desultory. Now, a couple of weeks before house officer jobs commenced, I found a post at Edendale, a district general hospital in a black township south of Pietermaritzburg. The job lacked academic prestige but I thought I'd be more comfortable away from the hierarchy of a teaching hospital. Also, I was happy to be back in Natal, for I'd missed its bush and grasslands. Pietermaritzburg was only about sixty miles from tropical Durban, where scents were stronger in the steamy air and the city's beaches and markets and sordid sailors' nightclubs were an invigorating contrast to Cape Town's rather self-aware gentility. Debra was still in the midst of her studies at

Cape Town University. She would be staying on in her swaying house among the Constantia pines. We made uncertain plans to see each other in the future.

☉

Pietermaritzburg was Natal's provincial capital. Its buildings were of weighty Victorian architecture, as perfectly preserved as the manners of its English settler population. At the start of the Zulu War of 1879 a red-coated British army had marched out of the town behind its regimental bands towards the Tugela River that formed the border with Zululand. Some days later an exhausted despatch rider had galloped into Pietermaritzburg with a tale of calamity: the entire central column of the invasion force had been wiped out at Isandhlwana, in the greatest defeat ever suffered by a modern army at the hands of 'savages'. By lantern-light an officer read out the names of the missing, many of them local men who had joined the force as scouts or as troopers with the Natal Mounted Police. The townspeople foresaw their imminent annihilation under Zulu spears. Buildings were fortified and the scholars of Pietermaritzburg Boy's High School issued with guns. The school tie – a wide band of black, a narrow one of white, and in between the thinnest line of red – commemorated this event in its history, and the cadet corps armoury still contained racks of Zulu War vintage Martini Henry rifles, cut down to schoolboy size, that were used for drill.

In fact the Zulu King Cetshwayo had had no intention of attacking the Natal colony. He'd still believed that the war could be stopped, and that the unmeetable terms of the ultimatum presented to him by the British colonial authorities had been a misunderstanding rather than a deliberate pretext for destroying his kingdom. But following the Isandhlwana debacle, fresh divisions from England and India were landed in Durban and the invasion re-launched. Resisting desperately, Cetshwayo's army was forced to retreat. In the final battle, at the royal kraal at Ulundi, his regiments were cut down as they charged against massed firepower. Cetshwayo's capital was put to the torch, its original site now marked by a dusty cemetery containing the graves of a dozen British dead, and a stone commemorating those tens of thousands of Zulu warriors who fell in defence of the Old Order and have no known resting place.

A few miles from the old battlefield lay the new town of Ulundi, now the capital of KwaZulu, the Zulu 'homeland'. The planners of Apartheid visualised a shining future when there would be no black South Africans; instead they would all be citizens of such homelands, whose passports they would carry (if they were ever allowed to travel) and whose tribal governments, appointed by Pretoria, would be responsible for their welfare. Economically 'unproductive' Zulus were expected to sustain themselves on the eroded soil of the overcrowded rural homeland, where malnutrition abounded. Those who found work dwelt in black townships situated around the margins of Natal's cities and industrial areas. These dormitory settlements, though distant from KwaZulu, were demarcated as parts of the homeland and administered by the KwaZulu government. The hospital in the white town of Pietermaritzburg, run by the Natal Provincial Administration, was modern, equipped to European standards, efficient and calm. Edendale Hospital, a few miles away, was the responsibility of the KwaZulu Ministry of Health and struggled to function far beyond capacity.

The hospital stood on a hill at the edge of the township, a six-floor tower of brown brick among wings and outbuildings. The doctors' quarters with their dining hall, billiard room and swimming pool lay at the back of the hospital. Being geographically in KwaZulu, South African laws such as the Group Areas Act did not apply, enabling us to live alongside doctors of other racial classifications – and share the same swimming pool – in a way that was entirely illegal in neighbouring white Pietermaritzburg. My black colleagues included the son of the Lesotho Minister of Health who had arranged for me to work in the country's Flying Doctor Service when I'd been a student. Beyond the hospital gates began the packed rows of houses roofed with tin, the unlicensed drinking places called *shebeens* whose dark interiors vented *kwela* music amplified to distortion and the smell of beer and dust. Long before dawn, the smoke of kitchen fires would fill the streets as people roused themselves to take the bus to work in distant factories. At night the residents stepped nervously between the occasional streetlights, fearful of gangster knifemen after their pay. From all this we lived in isolation, cut off by high security fences that enclosed the hospital grounds, and – by a slope of watered lawn and flower-beds – from our patients, crowded into the wards and clinics of the hospital buildings.

Though I'd worked on the 'non-white' wards of my Cape Town teaching hospital while a student, this was my first real experience of African medicine. I had responsibility for patients on a male and a female medical ward of mixed pathology, each holding around fifty beds. Pneumonia cases lay beside those with cardiac failure, amoebic liver abscesses or fits. The vast rooms smelt of Lifebuoy soap and the maize-meal porridge served to the patients from trundling cauldrons on wheels. There were no curtains that might have allowed for a measure of privacy; indeed, curtain-rails would have simply got in the way, for the beds were constantly in motion, either being pushed together to make space for new patients or, when beds ran out, being shifted apart to allow further admissions to occupy mattresses between them on the floor. A fragile screen might be found to partly hide someone undergoing an intimate procedure such as a rectal examination, and patients with contagious illnesses like typhoid or hepatitis would be isolated in a small side-room, but the general population of the wards suffered and socialised, and sometimes died, shoulder to shoulder.

The consultant physician under whom I worked was a farmer. Peterson drove to the hospital each morning in a truck loaded with maize. While he did ward-rounds, one of his workers ran a stall inside the hospital gates, grilling mielies and selling them to those queuing outside the outpatients department. Peterson wore a safari suit and suede *veldskoen* ankle boots and moved about the wards as he might walk his lands, chivvying and joking with the patients in fluent Zulu. Marshalled by the white-uniformed ward sister, her maroon epaulettes carrying the enamelled badges of her rank, the patients would be sitting up straight in bed with their folders placed at the corner of the red blanket. After an exchange of formal greetings Peterson would ask what had brought them to hospital and how they were getting on. From these exchanges I learned a vocabulary of Zulu anatomical and diagnostic terms regarding frequency and intensity of pain, bowel function, urination and breath, and – repeated over and over – the litany of questions needed to take a history from a potential TB case:

Uyakhwehlela? – Do you have a cough?

Uqalenini? – For how long?

Uyajuluga ebusuku? – Do you sweat at night?

Ukhwehlela igazi? – Are you coughing blood?

Tuberculosis accounted for many admissions, the disease flourishing in the dense overcrowding of the township and the workers' dormitories. It challenged every specialty in the hospital. Tuberculosis of the spine, hip and other bones formed a major part of the work of the orthopaedic department, the surgeons treated intestinal TB, and children with tuberculous meningitis were admitted under the paediatricians. Those on our adult wards generally had lung infection, though there were also some with kidney tuberculosis or ulcerated lymph nodes in the neck. The TB patients were kept together, quarantined in a special room at the end of the ward for an initial four-month course of daily tablets and injections. It was these patients Mrs Zondi, Mr Dhlamini, Miss Shabalala, *Mfundise* (Venerable) Zwelathini – who were the people I came to know best, greeting them each morning, enquiring after their progress and examining them using clinical methods that at medical school had seemed obscure and befuddling and were now revealed as essential diagnostic techniques. I percussed chests, tapping one middle finger with the other to detect the hollow note of cavities in the underlying lung or the dullness of accumulated fluid. Auscultation through my stethoscope revealed the harsh sigh of bronchial breathing conducted through fibrosis or solidified lung, the vibration called vocal resonance or that intimate clarity of sound known as whispering pectoriloquy.

With sixty or seventy patients under my care and every third night and weekend on call, I was learning to work hard. Ward rounds began before eight, followed by outpatient clinics where I'd see people with pneumonia or hypertension, coughing blood from TB, shitting blood from amoebic dysentery or pissing blood from schistosomiasis. Most attenders showed an extra-ordinary stoicism, coming to the hospital only if they believed they were going to die.

At night we'd be called to the emergency department to admit cases in diabetic crisis or with life-threatening asthma, and asked to assess obscure clinical problems; rigidity and staring eyes might be tetanus, catatonia, hysteria or meningitis. We also dealt with any problems arising on the wards.

One Saturday morning in the small hours I was dragged from an exhausted sleep by the chime of my pager, flashing an urgent summons to the male ward. Somnambulating, I threw on my white coat and staggered down the steps of the doctors' quarters into the warm, dew-wet night. Frogs barked in the valley below the swimming pool. In the tower only night-lights glimmered at the windows of the nurses' stations. Stumbling into the lift, I propped myself in a corner and knuckled the button for the top floor. The doors closed.

I was roused from my doze as the lift stopped suddenly and the lights went out. From the fan in the overhead vent came an extinguishing sigh. At once the pitch-dark air became stifling, loaded with the building's trapped heat. I fumbled for the control panel. A protruding knob caught my fingers and I slammed it in. Far away a bell began to trill, faint and ignorable, and now panic arrived, for I realised I had often heard that distant alarm, ringing unattended through the hospital for hours. I knew too that no engineer would be driving out from Pietermaritzburg into the township at this hour on a weekend; indeed, probably not till Monday morning. An asphyxiating terror crushed my chest and I flailed my fists against the invisible metal walls. After an immeasurable time, the lift lurched – up or down, I didn't know – and then a sliver of light appeared as the doors began to open. The floor-edge was almost at waist height but I dived through the gap and, picking myself up from the linoleum, tore down the stairs so fast that I was falling. Outside in the night air I filled my lungs like a man drowning.

Over the alarm bell's distant ring I realised that I was hearing another sound: my pager, still calling me to the ward with relentless urgency. I ran, taking the steps three at a time. Six floors up I rushed into the ward to be confronted by a scene that stopped me momentarily in my tracks. A bed had been rolled from its place into the pool of light outside the sister's office. In it a man sat forward, supported between a pair of nurses. His eyes fixed on me as I entered, and I recognised strong, dignified Mr Dhlamini, under my care for the past six weeks for pulmonary TB. Between his knees a steel basin slopped bloody froth. The man's lips and chin were glazed with bright blood that bubbled with each rattling breath; it was clear that the disease had eroded into a major pulmonary vessel.

'What's his blood pressure?' I asked the nurses and at once they vanished into the darkness, their heels clattering. I felt for his pulse. Dhlamini looked at me beseechingly. His mouth opened wider and there emerged a rush of blood, surging like a turned-on tap. Shouting for the nurses to come back, I drove the bed on its stiff castors to the suction unit on the wall, but it did not work and while I waited for them to find another one I held him on his side and tried to get a drip-needle into a vein in his neck and listened to him gurgling in his haemorrhage.

I don't know what I could have done if I'd arrived there sooner. An ideal outcome would have required a skilled thoracic surgeon waiting in the operating theatre to get Mr Dhlamini's chest open, dissect amidst matted, tubercular nodes in the lung-root to find the source of bleeding and tie it off. But such facilities were rare at any district general hospital, and unattainable in the middle of the night. The fluid we poured in through his drip-line ran out through his lungs at such a rate that the suction machine laboured in the flood. The oxygen mask bubbled, half submerged. Dhlamini's eyes lost focus and developed a distant, expectant look. His pulse became irregular, then stopped. The medical registrar turned up amidst the blood and mess in time to stop me electrocuting myself with the heart defibrillator. After certifying the time of death in the patient's notes, he led me off the ward. Numbly, I followed him until we reached the open doors of the lift, but I found myself unable to pass through them. From then on I took the stairs instead.

✪

Off-duty, the doctors' quarters offered little sanctuary from the pressures of the wards. A couple of the live-in registrars were scions of the great Natal sugar dynasty families. They had attended one of the province's exclusive boarding schools and affected rather patrician airs. One was in addition a Christian – though I saw no particular humility in his behaviour towards his patients – and would demand silence at the dining table to say grace. Other doctors were rugby players and held drunken parties on the weekends, which were attended by those prepared to venture into the township for a thrash: policemen, their lipstick-smothered girlfriends and younger sisters in excruciatingly tight jeans who smashed back brandy and Coke, vomited early and passed out on the grass by the poolside. Rowdy accidents involving broken glass were not uncommon, and the party had sometimes to adjourn to the casualty department for lacerations to be sutured. One of the doctors was notorious for his drinking – bottles of cane spirit downed-in-one for a dare – and would end the night comatose, being resuscitated though an intravenous drip.

I tried to get away from the hospital as much as possible. With fellow doctor Stu-ball, my good friend and ex-classmate from Cape Town, I'd go to more entertaining parties in Pietermaritzburg or to the drive-in cinema on the hill above the town, where mist blocked out the screen often enough to make it worthwhile bringing a book. Stu-ball invited me to move out of the hospital quarters and join him and a carpenter named Fred in a delightful old farmhouse on a hillside above Pietermaritzburg. It was reached via a track that snaked up through bush and overgrown orange groves, fording streams that foamed against the car-wheels in the rains. From the veranda that surrounded the house we looked over ornamental gardens run to seed, and groves of bamboo. The property backed onto a thousand acres of bush. Early each morning a troop of monkeys would swing through the garden, leaping one by one from the palms flanking the front steps to land with a thump on the sheet-iron roof of my bedroom.

Evenings that I was not on duty I'd shower off the miasma of the hospital, jump into my VW bus and drive through Pietermaritzburg to reach the freeway for Durban to visit my brother. Coming off the high plateau, the coastal lights spread below, I'd feel the air thicken with that familiar heat. We'd eat in seafood restaurants and go to student parties in big old houses full of surfers, revolutionaries, comic-strip artists, dope smokers and lively girls.

One invited me back to the house behind the Ridge that she shared with a group of militant lesbians. They had saved her from a previous unhappy heterosexual relationship and now beat on the door of her bedroom and demanded to know if we were having penetrative sex, an activity expressly forbidden by key articles of the household charter. Then there was no longer time to consider having affairs because I started paediatrics, working a one-in-two, which meant that every second evening and weekend I did not come home from the hospital but stayed on duty.

Children often came in severely ill. Unless treated promptly, they tended to die quietly and without fuss, for they did not struggle for life as we do when we are older, but relinquished it with a peculiar acceptance. Sometimes the pathology was obvious – breathless with pneumonia, dehydrated by gastroenteritis or convulsing from high fever – but often they would be simply listless and unresponsive and it would be essential to establish if any of these conditions was the cause, or whether they might in fact be suffering from meningitis. The younger they were, the less reliable were the key meningitis symptoms of neck stiffness and aversion to light, and it was practice to perform a lumbar puncture on almost all babies and children where there was diagnostic uncertainty. This exacting procedure, with its possible complications, initially terrified me, but I became adept at tapping cerebrospinal fluid from between the lumbar vertebrae with the first smooth slide of the needle. Holding the sample to the light, I could assess the cloudiness of a bacterial infection or the fine spider-webs of protein associated with tuberculosis and start treatment, even before the report arrived back from the lab.

Those with TB meningitis were hardest to treat. Some remained on the wards, brain-damaged and prone to prolonged seizures. Their mothers would sit at the foot of the cot, distraught and uncomprehending, leaping up at each ward round with an unreasoning hope while we tried – through the nursing sister – to comfort without giving false reassurance, for there was no treatment and no facility for long-term care and we were waiting for nature, in the form of a quiet pneumonia, to deal mercifully with the situation. Infections flourished on the ward. The whole time I worked there I suffered from some bug or other, caught via the coughs and sneezes of fifty tiny throats or – despite my ritualised hand-washing with iodine soap – communicated from their guts to mine. Scabies burrowed between my fingers, my lungs coughed green phlegm and bouts of diarrhoea wrung me dry.

My second month on the paediatric ward coincided with an epidemic of gastroenteritis. Babies arrived, heads lolling, eyes sunk back, their skin dry and sagging from fluid loss. The only sign of life would be a heartbeat fluttering between the birdlike fragility of the ribs. The neon-lit rehydration ward contained no cots, just a waist-high counter along the walls on which the babies were laid. From a wire overhead were suspended bags of intravenous fluid, and the fine tubing of the giving-sets hung down in the greenish light like aerial roots in a long herbarium. Often the only place that it was possible to find a vein was on the scalp. I would shave soft hair from the temples and place a rubber band around the head as a tourniquet to show the vessel, no thicker than a thread, that I was hoping to cannulate. Advancing the needle with tiny probings, I'd sense the resistance of skin and fascia and hope to feel the tiny tick as it entered the vein. Success was marked by a strand of blood, dark and sluggish, curling back into the plastic tube, and I'd tape the drip in place and start it going, counting the drops as they fell through the clear chamber to establish that the flow-rate was correct. Sometimes, for an instant, I'd remember counting drops in Israel, a child myself, and then I'd slide the baby along the counter – the drip-bag accompanying it on the overhead wire – and turn to the next.

The paediatric wards looked like a gypsy encampment. Mothers from the township wore the head-scarves and uniforms of domestic workers, or their Sunday best with a Zionist Church badge; those from rural villages might be blanket-wrapped, in strings of beadwork. During the day they sat beside their children's places; at night, wrapping cloths around their heads, they occupied mats laid on the floor of the wards and the lift lobby and the corridor, so that we picked our way from patch to patch of linoleum like stepping-stones between the sleepers. The population of the ward changed constantly. Babies, near to death one day, might be bright-eyed and happy the next, bundles of such beauty that they melted the hearts of even the staunchest racists on the staff.

'*Ag,* but these little ones is *lekker,*' said a thickset Afrikaner registrar, dandling an infant on his knee. 'What a pity they grow up to be so horrible.'

✛

There followed my mandatory stint in the hospital's anaesthetics department, during which I had to carry out inductions on fifty patients, a requirement of the South African Medical Council to prepare all doctors for possible work in rural areas. My lessons from Mercier in the Seychelles served me well, for he had taught me how to make people unconscious and to intubate and ventilate them, but I hadn't appreciated the cumulative effect of breathing exhaled anaesthetic gasses day and night as I sat by the heads of my patients. In the stillness of the operating theatres, with few distractions but the repetitive recording of blood pressure and pulse and the ventilator's slow wheeze, my own level of consciousness fluctuated in inverse ratio to that of my charge and I understood why surgeons referred to their anaesthetic colleagues, with dry humour, as 'the half-asleep looking after the half-awake'.

Diversions, when they came, were usually unwanted – a patient failing to start breathing again or a dropping blood pressure from surgical bleeding – or merely unpleasant, such as the stink from drainage of a foetid abscess. I was watching a surgeon carrying out this operation on a humid midnight when something splashed in the steel bowl that was collecting the pink-and-custard swirls of pus. Squatting in the broth was a small brown frog that looked back at me before springing upward, planting a pus-print on the cap of the astonished nurse and bouncing away to a corner of the operating theatre. I looked for it on the floor and saw that it had landed among hundreds of others; a plague of frogs, hatched as though by the night's heat. The sister seized a mop and tried to sweep them to the door, triggering a frenzy of jumping that filled the room with bouncing shapes. They landed on the drapes, in the wound, and on the gowns and gloves. All semblance of sterility was lost.

The world seemed to be tending to increasing instability. One afternoon a tornado appeared out of nowhere. In the outpatients department we'd noticed the changing light through the windows and the sky turn a brassy brown. Doors banged as people who'd been queuing outside dashed in for shelter, then the wind struck the building with such force that the walls rang. Nothing was visible beyond the glass but a deluge of water through which objects appeared briefly. Sheets of roofing from the garages cartwheeled by. Tree branches and guttering, even individual bricks, sailed past horizontally. The flat roof of the outpatients unit – a long building of prefabricated construction – began to undulate, showing glimpses of light at one corner. Inside, rain lashed us and papers swirled in the air. The storm passed in minutes, leaving the hospital grounds ankle-deep in freezing water and drifts of bricks from the disintegrated garages.

Outside the hospital, the war I'd foreseen in my childhood seemed to be coming home. The papers ran scare-stories about ANC battalions being infiltrated into the country to commence the 'Total Onslaught'. Convoys of armoured police Casspirs roared along the Durban highway and soldiers manned roadblocks at the off-ramps to the townships in night-time security actions. Nearing Pietermaritzburg at four one morning, my truck losing momentum up a long hill, I saw a set of headlights appear over the crest ahead and approach at high speed on my side of the highway. Behind it on the skyline materialised the flashing blue lights of pursuing police vans. Their quarry, a big sedan, swooped towards me and I tugged the wheel desperately to avoid its path. Then it leaned the other way without slackening speed and ploughed a long diagonal across the grass of the central reservation until its wheels jammed in a stormdrain. The cops pulled up alongside my stopped truck and opened fire with rifles, as though on a shooting range, at the figures scattering from the juddering vehicle. At the hospital next day I found one of their targets lying in the intensive care unit after surgery: a fourteen-year-old boy who'd been shot through the chest and abdomen.

✛

I needed a break from Edendale. Debra came up from Cape Town to see me, and I took some leave in order that we might resurrect our relationship. We decided to make a visit northwards to see my friend David, doing his house officer year at a township hospital outside Bulawayo, Rhodesia's second city. A 'terrorist war' had been under way in Rhodesia for the past eight years. I'd never visited the country, but there'd been a lot of Rhodesians at Cape Town University, which they considered a sort of spiritual home. The campus had been built on land donated by Cecil John Rhodes and a great granite-pillared memorial to the arch-imperialist stood on the mountainside above, with a bronze figure – 'this vast and brooding spirit,' according to Kipling's epitaph – gazing northwards over an Empire that he'd intended should extend from the Cape to Cairo. The Rhodesian Students Society was active on campus, with a notice board (headed 'Rhodesia is Super') announcing social events and carrying photographs of white youths in camouflage shirts and tight little shorts posing in front of the bodies of dead 'terrs'. There was also the odd official declaration:

> Fellow Rhodesians, our President has called upon us to pray for the nation, for deliverance from our enemies. In our situation, in Rhodesia today, those enemies are:
>
> 1. The International Communist Conspiracy;
> 2. The unrighteous double standards of the United Nations and the World Council of Churches;
> 3. The fifth column propagators of permissiveness in morality, pornography and drug addiction within our land;
> 4. And finally, the grass roots apathy about our situation and about God.

Debra and I drove north in my VW bus, carrying supplies – a dozen bottles of spirits – that we'd heard were scarce in that blockaded country. South Africa was defying UN sanctions, allowing the passage of ammunition, spare parts and fuel, but they couldn't send any heavy matériel; it was all needed for their own war in Angola. Rhodesians had responded to the embargo with great inventiveness. They'd modified commercial vehicles for military use, mobilised every aircraft in the country – including a World War Two Spitfire – and even made 'whisky' and 'gin' from sugar-cane spirit, but the genuine article was greatly in demand. At the bridge over the Limpopo that formed the border crossing, the Rhodesian customs officers were bemused but welcoming. They found it strange that we should come as casual visitors, for tourists were a rarity in these troubled times, but they pressed on us extra books of petrol coupons and warm wishes for our stay.

'Tell them Down South how well we're doing,' they said, 'Tell them we're prepared to go all the way.'

That night we laagered in the grounds of the Beit Bridge Motel, which was surrounded by barbed wire. The other guests appeared to be South African businessmen, on their way to meetings in Bulawayo and Salisbury. Embargo-breakers – traders in tyres, security accessories and family handguns – they were accompanied by their teenage sons, with whom they got drunk beside the motel swimming pool.

'Where's our beers, you stupid munt?' a down-cheeked eighteen-year-old yelled at an elderly back waiter. He turned for the approval of his father. 'How can these people expect to run a country if they can't even get our drinks right?'

Early the next morning we joined the other travellers at the sandbagged checkpoint on the edge of town, to be addressed by the Convoy Officer. Despite bullish government communiqués, the Rhodesian forces had by now lost control of much of the countryside to the guerrillas. The only way to travel on the roads was in convoy, with armoured cars at the front and rear of the column. These precautions did not prevent regular ambushes, so drivers had to be briefed on what to do in case of an attack. The officer, a white-haired police reservist, explained the tactics.

'If you hear shooting, just drive like hell. Don't stop for anything – someone waving you down, an overturned car – anything at all. Just put your head flat on the accelerator and go go go. The army's right behind you, and we'll pick up the pieces.'

He ordered a weapons check. I noticed that the businessmen wore pistols strapped below their bulging bellies. Some brought submachine guns from their briefcases and cocked them ostentatiously. Automatic rifles were produced from the trunks of cars. I stood with my hands in my pockets.

'Where's your weapon?' enquired the officer.

'I, er, don't have one,' I answered. 'I'll rely on the head-on-the-accelerator technique.'

The man regarded me stonily.

'You don't always have the choice, sonny. If you're white you're the enemy, and you better be ready to shoot. I'll give you a trooper, to ride up front in your VW.' He indicated a soldier in camouflage uniform standing nearby. 'You'll be doing him a favour, because he's off home on leave. And he'll be doing you a favour by giving you some firepower. You'd better bring your fuck-truck to the front, directly behind the lead gunship. You're the biggest target, so we'll put you in the most secure place in the convoy.'

We rolled off along the pocked tar road, following a drab-painted pickup. A rotating mount on its rear carried a heavy machine gun, shielded by steel plate. A man, strapped into the firing-seat, swung the weapon round and back as he scanned the passing bush. Behind us stretched the long train of the convoy, each car a porcupine of protruding gun barrels. It felt anything but secure. By this stage of the war every white Rhodesian male from eighteen to fifty-five was being called up, alternating forty-eight days in the forces with forty-eight days out. Our soldier had just completed a stint in the bush and he was jumpy with nerves and exhaustion. He sat wedged against the passenger door, smoking tremulously, his weapon stuck out of the window. The day before, his leave due, he had hitched a ride in from the operational area with a couple of army trucks coming to Beit Bridge to collect rations. He'd been in the second vehicle when, on a bush track, the lead truck had gone over a mine.

'The back was full of empties, man, crates of Coke bottles. The whole lot blew upward.' He lifted his hands, then dropped them onto his thighs. 'There were three troopies riding on top of the load. They were completely fucked.'

I approached a bend and accelerated to catch up with the gun-truck, momentarily out of sight ahead.

'Jesus Christ,' the man screamed, racking a shell into the chamber of his automatic rifle. 'Slow down, slow down!'

He hunched around the gun, peering into the high grass. Abruptly he slapped the dashboard: 'Go quickly, let's get out of here,' and I floored the pedal.

'Sorry, man,' he gasped, lighting another cigarette, 'that's just the sort of place they hit you. I get really frightened when I can't see around the corner.'

Bulawayo was stifling, an embattled city. Angular armoured trucks growled along the boulevards. Department stores and cinemas had checkpoints where bags were searched for bombs. With many doctors away 'on ops' my friend David was working almost constantly, and I hardly saw him. Debra and I decided to drive out from Bulawayo to the Matopo Hills, a range of granite domes that bulged up out of the veld thirty miles to the southwest. Cecil John Rhodes used to come to the highest of these outcrops and gaze out from the top, contemplating his domain; his remains were interred in a grave cut into his lookout point under a brass plate. At the police checkpoint on the edge of Bulawayo the officer told us to be careful, 'terrorist infiltrators' had been reported in the area, but an army sweep had so far yielded nothing. Normally he would have stopped us going, he said, but as we were so keen to visit Rhodes's grave... We drove along the empty road that shimmered in the morning sun.

A bullet-punctured signboard marked the turn-off to the sacred mountain. Army trucks were parked in the picnic area and a rifle-toting black trooper led us up the curved shoulder of the rock to the top. An officer, standing at the grave site, scanned the lands around through binoculars. As we returned to the VW we met a Rhodesian family in the car park, starting their pilgrimage. Father wore a pistol and a black nanny carried a toddler. The mother pushed a high-wheeled pram, which a baby shared with an automatic rifle.

A few miles further along the Matopos road we pulled off at a signpost indicating a site of Bushman paintings. Debra and I waded across a stream and climbed the path to an overhanging ledge, where ghostly ochre antelope filed past stick-figure hunters. In a sun-warmed hollow we took off our clothes and made love. The sound of an aircraft made us look up. Directly above us a small green spotter plane wobbled on the updrafts, its pilot bellowing down to us through a megaphone over the engine's drone. '...back to your vehicle,' he shouted, '... back to town ... army's called in a contact ... not safe.'

Nearing Bulawayo, we offered a lift to some black people waiting at the roadside for a bus. The police at the next checkpoint, glancing at my South African number plates, waved me through. I was aware of my silent cargo crouched on the floor behind my seat as I accelerated past lines of Africans being body-searched against the stopped buses. Others sat on the verge, hands clasped on their heads, under the muzzle of a machine gun. As we picked up speed I heard whispers, then laughter, from my relieved passengers.

'Thank you, brother,' came a voice. 'Thanks to you we shall see our families tonight.'

It was so easy just then to see the issue clearly. Simply by being there, I had helped these people. The gesture was tiny, in the face of all the difficulties they endured, yet it had been something. Full of a joy of belonging, I dropped them off at the township where they lived.

The feeling did not survive dinner. David had been invited to the house of colleagues and brought us along. Sitting on the patio, sipping drinks (our gift of gin and whisky having been gratefully received), Debra and I told the story of our *al fresco* love-making at the Matopos, and the arrival of the spotter aircraft. Buoyed up by the amusement with which it was received, I mentioned too the happiness I had felt on helping my passengers get past the police post. The mood of the party darkened at once.

'What if those had been terrorists smuggling grenades into the city?' demanded a young mother, breathless with hysteria.

'They weren't,' I answered. 'They were just ordinary people trying to get home.'

'You South Africans don't understand how serious things are,' said an exhausted-looking doctor. 'You wait until it starts happening down there.'

6

Homicide

I'd grown up with a story of my father's about being in England in 1945, just after the war in Europe had ended. Waiting to be demobilised, he was surviving on his officer's pay while finding a hospital post and preparing for the examination of Fellowship of the Royal College of Surgeons, though he'd been able to put away his uniform when a suit was sent out to him by his mother in South Africa. London 'society' had survived the war, and despite rationing and bomb damage was managing to maintain certain standards. Being presentably attired and well brought up, my dad was taken by another Royal College of Surgeons candidate to a dinner party at a fashionable address in Knightsbridge. They'd arrived at the house, handed their overcoats to the manservant and been shown through to the drawing room, where – with the curtains closed against the rainy night outside – there was light and gaiety and no depressing military colours to be seen.

The pleasant impression persisted as they went through to dinner, where my father found himself seated beside an attractive young woman. Conversation was sparked by two obvious talking-points: a chandelier over the dining table that had belonged to actress Lily Langtree, mistress of King Edward VII; and the entrée, a delicacy unseen since the war's start – shrimp on a bed of fluffy white rice – obtained by the host from an American officer with connections in the Pacific Theatre of Operations. Chatter flowed up and down the table and glasses were refilled, but my father was having difficulties with one of his shrimp. It curled around his tongue, his molars bouncing from its leathery resilience. He brought a covert hand to his mouth and tugged at the hard bit of shell at the tail, but it would not detach. Without attracting attention, my father deposited the mouthful in his napkin and replaced it on his lap, where, after a minute or two, he was able to steal a peep between the folds. The object in the napkin was a yellowish human finger, the nail still attached.

'The little finger of some poor rice-picker,' he'd say, to our shocked exclamations, 'or a fisherman's. I couldn't ruin the party for everyone else – the meal was a luxury, after years of whale meat – so I stuck the napkin in my pocket and excused myself. In the bathroom I flushed away the finger, then went back to the table. I never told anybody about it at the time because it would have appeared an affront to one's hosts, and etiquette is so important to the English. Besides, I did quite hope to see that girl again.'

I'd wondered if being in the war did that to you; put you on such familiar terms with death that you could tolerate the thought of its finger down your throat. At Cape Town medical school, during my training in forensic pathology, I'd been repelled and horrified by the enamel trays of dissociated body parts that sometimes greeted us at the police mortuary on a Monday morning. The painted toenails on a waxy foot, a jaw fresh-shaven, with good teeth but no head, were evidence of a violent disruption of life by incomprehensible forces that made me fear for my own existence. The mortuary housed a small forensic museum in which we could open the display cases and handle the exhibits. Considering the high-velocity gunshot wounds being dealt out in the townships by the police and army, and the caches of 'communist' rocket-propelled grenades that the government displayed as proof of the terrorist menace, the items in the museum were downright quaint. Sealed glass dishes held old cartridges – rim-fire and pin-fire, obsolete a century before – arrayed on cotton poufs. There were daggers taken from sailors at the docks and a rusty 'opera pistol' with a folding trigger. Files contained photographs of bodies: found immersed in water, in dry rooms, stewed in the sun, and the differing characteristics of their forms of decomposition – saponification, mummification, liquefactive necrosis – a gallery of the monstrous transformations wrought by death.

Some of these items were used for questions in our forensic practical examination. A knife was shown alongside a picture of a wound and an opinion requested about whether the evidence matched. There was a skull with a hole punched through it that exactly fitted the steel core of the stiletto heel on a red shoe: could this have been the murder weapon? Colour images of empurpled corpses were shown, inviting us to state whether the appearances were those of post-mortem lividity or carbon monoxide poisoning. I hadn't done adequate preparation for the test, imagining that some intuitive, investigative flair would reveal the answers, but my poor showing was made clear by the fact that I was among the rump of also-ran candidates interviewed in pairs at the oral examination. The professor started with my classmate, a sweet girl who clearly found the subject of violent death appropriately distasteful. After struggling to find an area of forensic pathology in which he could elicit from her even a molecule of knowledge, he put to her what might have been his rock-bottom reserve question.

'So,' he asked, 'how would you kill someone if you didn't want to be found out?'

After the man had pointed out the glaring evidence associated with her suggestion of suffocation by pillow, he turned to me. I was determined to elude detection for a little longer and came out with the perfect murder as once suggested by my erudite friend Graeme: exposing the victim to a tasteless, colourless, unlikely–to–be suspected organic poison – later actually used by a special South African covert military unit as an assassination method – that would bring about delayed death by irreversible organ failure. The examiner squinted at me speculatively, for long enough that I wondered if I was being considered for academic distinction, but he gave me a Third. At least I'd passed.

✛

At the end of my house-officer posts at hospitals in Edendale and Cape Town, I'd been called up for the army. Like my father, I had elected not to serve the South African Defence Force in its current conflict, and was instead following in his academic footsteps: thirty-five years after he'd arrived in England at the end of his wartime service, I was sitting in a wood-panelled lecture theatre in London, attending a preparatory course for the primary examination of the

Fellowship of the Royal College of Surgeons. The professor of anatomy had elucidated the muscle compartments of the forearm, and the relations of nerve branches to arteries where they lay between the bones. Now, in the last minute before time was up, he mentioned the method used to identify which hand a detached finger had come from. Hairs on the backs of the fingers grow pointing outwards, he told us, so that on the left hand they point to the left and on the right hand to the right; a useless bit of knowledge until he'd had to go one night during the London Blitz into an underground shelter in Piccadilly Circus to try to establish the number of people disintegrated by the direct hit of a five-hundred-kilogram German bomb.

Finding a London hospital post had been reasonably straight-forward – the levels of responsibility required of us as junior hospital doctors in South Africa meant that we could manage most clinical situations with reasonable confidence – but my colonial origins were not appreciated by everyone. This was made evident at an interview for a post at a prestigious London teaching hospital. The panel had seemed satisfied by my answers regarding my experience and ability, and now deferred to the senior consultant, a pinstripe-suited public school type with prodigious, rust-coloured eyebrows.

'South African, eh?' he gurgled, staring at me down his nose. 'Tell meh; are yaw plenning to stay in the United Kingdom?'

'Yes.'

'Reallah.' His throat constricted further in a spasm of disapproval. 'Hev yaw considahd tekking elocution lessons?'

I'd arrived in England at a grim time. The elevation of Margaret Thatcher as prime minister appeared to have unleashed some deep meanness, an upsurge of selfishness and institutionalised brutality. I noticed how ready the police were to put the boot in, as measured by the incidence of prisoners brought to the casualty department bruise-faced, half throttled, with handcuffs ratcheted to the tightest, wrist-fracturing notch. Things back in South Africa were getting worse too. Buildings blazed in the townships on the BBC evening news, Casspirs rolled and police volleys felled stone-throwing black children. International momentum was building towards the imposition of economic sanctions against South Africa. Prime Minister Thatcher decried sanctions. What I wanted was to find sanctuary, keep below the sight-line of the UK authorities, and learn surgery. Instead I was having to remember my forensic toxicology.

Working as a senior house officer in orthopaedics, I admitted a patient with acute low back pain to my ward one weekend morning. He was a muscular, square-faced man with a brisk manner, who described his profession as 'civil servant'. After taking a medical history and examining him, I prescribed a muscle relaxant and pain relief and applied spinal traction. On my round that evening I asked him how he was getting on. He answered with difficulty, through a mouth so dry that his lips were sticking to his teeth. My patient complained of a raging thirst that several refills of his bedside water jug had been unable to assuage. Re-examination revealed a fever and clinical signs of dehydration. Puzzled, I took blood for further tests and started an intravenous infusion, placing a catheter in his bladder to measure urine output. The teaspoonful that emerged I took to the laboratory with the blood samples and asked the technician to expedite the man's results.

When I returned to the bedside a visitor was with him, a man of similar manner and build, whom I ushered out before addressing my patient.

'The blood results show a rather strange picture. The urea and electrolyte levels, and the analysis of liver function, suggest that your liver and kidney cells have been affected by something, perhaps a toxin. Have you been exposed to any chemical compounds?'

'Chemical compounds?' The man's tongue clicked on his parched palate. 'What sort of thing do you mean?'

'I'm not sure. Industrial solvents? Cleaning agents? Medication?'

My patient thought for a moment. 'Could chemical components of explosives cause it?'

'I suppose they could. But how would you be coming into contact –'

He raised a hand. 'I wonder if you could ask my visitor to come in, and leave us alone for a moment.'

Behind the screen the two men began to converse in low voices. I was in the ward sister's office, dialling the National Poisons Information Laboratory, when the visitor tapped on the glass.

'We need to talk to you.'

My patient stared at the ceiling. 'Ed isn't quite a straightforward civil servant,' explained the other man. 'He's a senior officer in the Scotland Yard anti-terrorism unit. I work with him. For the last few weeks we've been searching across London for bomb-factories, in warehouses and cellars.'

'Perhaps it's an infection, then,' I offered. 'Leptospirosis, caught from rat's urine.'

'But you said it could be from chemicals or explosives,' said the visitor.

'I was about to put out a call for the duty medical registrar. Hepato-renal failure isn't exactly an orthopaedic problem.'

The man shook his head. 'Better if you don't make any calls for the moment. I'll get someone to call you.'

A short time later the switchboard notified me of an incoming call.

'Evening, Doctor,' said a deep voice. 'Dr Inaudible speaking, Home Office pathologist. I hear you've got one of our chaps there. Give me a run-down of your findings.'

I described the clinical signs and the blood test results. I also told him that, despite the instructions I'd been given, I had involved the medical registrar, whose consultant was on his way in to the hospital; perhaps he would be the best person to talk to.

'We'll stick with you for the moment, old chap,' he said cheerily. 'Back to you in a little while.'

The phone in my duty room rang at two A.M. and another Dr Inaudible introduced himself.

'Calling from the Defence Medical Laboratory at Porton Down,' he announced. 'What are the latest blood results on our friend?'

When I'd finished listing them he thought for a while, making ruminative sounds as though sucking a caramel.

'What do you know about Ricin poisoning?' he asked.

By chance, I'd talked recently to a South African friend making a TV documentary about Georgi Markov, a Bulgarian exile working at the BBC who'd been killed by Ricin. The substance had been contained in a tiny steel pellet, injected into Markov's thigh at a London bus stop by an assassin using a specially modified umbrella.

'It's an organic toxin, from the castor oil seed. Fatal in very small doses, liver and kidney failure.'

'Indeed. Well, thanks, Doctor.'

I reached the ward for my morning round just as Ed was being hoisted onto a trolley by an ambulance crew for transfer to a specialist unit. He shook my hand. 'Thanks for your care. There's someone here to talk to you.'

A grey-haired man in a suit took me aside.

'Ricin,' he began. 'How do you come know about such an obscure poison?'

I repeated my incidental knowledge of the Markov case. The man wrote in his notebook.

'Ed was the Chief Inspector in the Markov investigation,' he said. 'He delivered the pellet to the Porton Down laboratory. Do you think he could have absorbed the stuff through his skin?'

'It's really not my field, but I imagine he would have to have handled it directly. Surely the thing was transported wrapped and sealed?'

The man made another note.

'Did anyone unknown to you come onto the ward?' he asked. 'We have to consider whether he could somehow have been poisoned once already in hospital.'

'Not that I can recall,' I said, and then, anxiously: 'I suppose you'd consider me a suspect, then?'

'Not at all.' He shut the book with a snap. 'Of course, we've checked up on you.'

✪

While I hauled myself up step after step of my surgical training, drowning in hospital work for up to a hundred hours a week, things were happening in the world I used to know. At the start of the 1980s, with international sanctions choking South Africa's oil supply, ANC guerrillas blew up the strategic synthetic oil refinery at Sasolburg and black smoke marred the pure Highveld sky. Even with the country's security forces fully deployed, the tide of insurgency and sabotage grew, with assaults on police stations, transport links, power stations and military installations. Rhodesia had become Zimbabwe, under black majority rule, and South Africa now faced infiltration along this border as well as those with Angola and Mozambique. Desperate to redress their loss of allies in the region, the South African National Intelligence Service (NIS) gave the go-ahead for a coup in the Seychelles that would put Jimmy Mancham back in power.

The operation was to be funded by a group of *Grand Blancs* who'd joined Sir James in exile, using a force of serving South African military personnel and private adventurers led by the mercenary Mike Hoare. The conspirators had assured Hoare that his arrival would spark a spontaneous uprising by the Seychellois people, 'oppressed beyond endurance', meantime beating down his fee from five million to one million and finally to three hundred thousand dollars. 'Mad Mike' agreed eventually to the tactically and financially risky plan of using a skeleton squad who would be paid on the successful toppling of René's government. The operation was launched in November 1981. Wearing matching blazers that identified them as a sports team called the Ancient Order of Froth-blowers, and with automatic rifles hidden in their kit-bags, the small assault force touched down at the airport in Mahé.

I could imagine them walking across the concrete towards that white terminal building, enfolded by the scented dusk, but I only found out what had happened next when I met one of the participants, twenty years later, in a bar in Durban. Duffy was a press photographer who'd once served in 5 Commando, Major Hoare's old Congo mercenary unit. He'd been recruited by the NIS for a sidebar to the Seychelles coup plan, to get into the Russian Embassy in Port Victoria during the confusion and photograph all the documents. Duffy told me the story as we drove around Durban in his little red van, looking for a photo location that he needed.

'We'd been told that ninety percent of Seychellois were members of the Seychelles People's Resistance and that all we had to do was hold the Tanzanian soldiers in their barracks beside the airport and the SPR would take over,' he explained. 'We had bad intelligence. The customs men were all supposed to be SPR, but they searched our luggage and found a guy's gun and started yelling, so we took over the terminal building and the control tower and then tried to go for the barracks. We'd been told that all their weapons were kept locked in the armoury and the Tanzanians were unarmed, but they had guns, all right, and an armoured car that we didn't know about – bad intelligence, you see – and they had us pinned down.

'So it's dark now and they're shooting the control tower to shit with this 12.7 in a sandpit at the end of the runway that we also didn't know about 'cos our intelligence was deficient, and more of them are shooting up the airport building and it's clear we're not going to get out of there, and suddenly there's this Air India passenger flight circling, requesting permission to land because the runway lights aren't on. We switch them on and as they come in the Tanzanians think it's reinforcements and open up on the plane with the 12.7 and miss with every round. So we take the plane and come home and hand back our weapons for which we'd had to indent from the South African military in the first place, and Mike says, 'Arrest some foreigners, blame them.' They held us for ten days and let us go, and we schemed that's all there was to it.'

I wasn't surprised that Duffy and the others had expected to get away scot-free; the South African Minister of Police, when questioned at the time in parliament about the Seychelles coup attempt, had replied, 'All they did was run around in the bush and break a few windows. Tell me what law they broke in South Africa.'

There was the awkward matter of a number of mercenaries and a South African NIS operative left behind in Seychelles when the plane took off. They were facing trial in Port Victoria, but here Margaret Thatcher's government had proved helpful, with solicitor Nicholas Fairburn MP – until recently a member of her parliamentary cabinet – made available to defend them in the Seychelles High Court. Eventually, though, international scorn had forced the South African authorities to take action.

'So a month later I'm sitting at home,' continued Duffy, 'and they come and arrest us for grabbing the plane. I remember they charged me with "man-stealing" – that's the Afrikaans for kidnapping – and all I said was, "Can't you change the wording a bit, that's going to look shit on my CV." I mean, I'd been hired for the job by the National Intelligence Service, so I never thought it would stick. I did two years.'

Duffy had been talking as he drove; now his car approached a military checkpoint set up on the Durban street. He began to steer the vehicle around the lanes of traffic cones. A soldier in full combat gear jumped out and raised his weapon to stop us, the rifle barrel wavering around the window edge.

'*Daily News!*' barked Duffy like a drill sergeant. 'Inform your senior officer.'

The soldier snapped to attention. Duffy crashed the van into gear and roared off. He chuckled. 'Should have known about that roadblock, we're doing a piece on the operation in tonight's paper. Bad intelligence.'

✪

Mike Hoare's calamitous coup attempt had happened as I was entering my third English winter. I thought of Godwin and Jo, sitting on their terrace listening to the BBC World Service in the warm evening. The Seychelles seemed a long way away. Despite the time I'd spent in London, the walls of my flat were bare as though I'd be leaving any day. But I couldn't return to the country of my birth, from where came reports of continuing tragedy. I was swallowing a sandwich one day in the doctors' lounge of my hospital when on the TV set a familiar face appeared: Neil, the trade union doctor with whom I'd shared a student house in Cape Town and last seen on his rustic farm outside Johannesburg, when I'd dropped off his girlfriend Liz. I leapt for the volume control.

'... is reported to have died in police custody. An enquiry, demanded by his family, has been refused. Friends and colleagues claim he was a victim of over-vigorous interrogation like the black student leader Steve Biko, who died five years ago of head injuries incurred during police questioning...'

The other doctors, their conversation interrupted, stared at me.

'I knew him,' I said, and they turned away and continued talking.

The bad news kept coming. In September 1984 the black townships around Johannesburg exploded with redoubled violence and the uprising spread across the country, despite the large-scale mobilisation of the army reserve to try to suppress it. Black rallies were met by gunfire, each fatality sparking more demonstrations and more deaths, and images of flames and armoured vehicles and bodies in the streets filled the BBC evening news. A state of emergency was declared. Jacqui, Debra's sister whom I'd admired and with whom I'd sometimes sparred, had returned to her teaching job in Lesotho. There she'd met and fallen in love with Joe, a member of the ANC, and they'd had a child. One evening in December 1985 a South African police hit-squad crossed the Caledon River into Lesotho – possibly over the unguarded drift near the motel we'd used to stay in – and were guided by an informer to a Maseru house where an ANC meeting was under way. The gunmen swept through the building, killing everyone inside. Joe had left the meeting early in order to help Jacqui prepare a party for their daughter's first birthday; now the killers were led to Joe's house. Once the neighbours were sure that the gunmen had gone, they entered the scene of carnage. Only the baby survived; screaming in her cot, splashed with her parents' blood.

☉

Neil and Jacqui had stayed to play their part, while I had left. Now they were dead who'd been so alive, so committed, and I, still alive, felt extinguished in the barrenness of exile. It was increasingly difficult to get news from home. In June 1986 the South African government extended the state of emergency to cover the media. Reporting of security force activity was banned and foreign journalists deported. The shootings, marches and detentions continued but there were no TV cameras to see them, and without visuals, the story faded from the international news.

By now a Fellow of the Royal College of Surgeons, I'd advanced up the surgical specialisation ladder and was equipped to perform the tasks expected of a surgical senior registrar: gastrectomies, colectomies, mastectomies. I had also trained in arterial surgery, spending hours joining blood vessels with tiny sutures, regular as a sewing machine. The youthful dreams of travel and commitment that had led me to enter medical school seemed remote, foolish, lost beneath the pervasive pressures of hospital existence. Even the relevant areas of my training had lagged. As a junior doctor in Cape Town I had dealt with mass casualties from police gunfire. Now the bloodshed and death was happening far away, and I wondered how I'd cope if faced with similar demands on my skills.

I'd returned from two research years in the US for a master's degree in surgery and was working as an air ambulance doctor while lining up my next hospital post when, in August 1990, Saddam Hussein invaded Kuwait. While an Allied military coalition was assembled and UN resolutions passed demanding Saddam's withdrawal – he promised to go when Israel obeyed the UN resolutions ordering it to withdraw from occupied Palestine – the British government was increasingly concerned about the presence of a number of its nationals hiding in Kuwait City. A network of private and Defence Ministry companies including British Aerospace, International Military Sales and Westland Helicopters had for years been selling military matériel to Saudi Arabia, Iraq, Kuwait and the other Gulf States under UK government Export Credit Guarantees; Saddam Hussein had been allowed to run up an overdraft of a billion pounds, making the British government a major investor in the fortunes of Iraq's ruler. Now senior officials in these companies, plus diplomatic staff – some of both also being 'assets' of the British military and intelligence services – needed to be brought home, not least because of the embarrassment should the West's role in supporting Saddam be revealed.

The phone rang one evening and a voice I didn't know asked for me by name. He had, the man explained, a proposition to discuss; nothing binding or definite, and it might be that nothing would come of it. He spoke with a slight stutter that hinted at an endearing diffidence, as though this were a person one could trust. I indicated my preparedness to listen. An operation was being considered, he continued, to extract some persons from Kuwait City. They would be brought by Kuwaiti helpers out into the desert, where 'security operatives' would guide them to a location for extraction by helicopter. A doctor with air-ambulance and surgical experience was needed to accompany the airborne evacuation in case there were injured among the group who needed treatment.

'You have been suggested as a possible candidate for the job,' he said. 'Think about it. We'll get back to you if it proceeds.'

In November there was a brief dip in tension. Saddam made a conciliatory announcement that his 'foreign guests' could leave, and a few days later I received a short call from the same voice saying that the operation was being stood down and thanking me for my 'interest'.

January 1991 saw a devastating campaign of aerial bombing launched on Baghdad and against Saddam's military forces along the Kuwaiti border. Six weeks later the Allied ground assault ripped through the under-equipped Iraqis, leaving a hundred thousand of them dead. I saw service after all. When the fighting ended with Saddam still in power, the Kurds in the north and the Shi'a in the south had – at the instigation of the West – launched an uprising against the dictator, only to be left to face the tanks and gunships of his Republican Guard. At the start of April I crossed the mountains into northern Iraq to work as a surgeon, treating wounded Kurdish *pesh merga* fighters. I operated in a forward position, a fort a couple of hundred yards behind the Kurdish front line. Gunfire and screaming would herald the arrival of wounded fighters, carried on a comrade's back, and I'd lay out my instruments and prepare the drugs; as the only doctor, I had not only to perform the surgery but to anaesthetise my patients beforehand.

There was little rest, for anyone turning up at the fort injured, unwell or simply requiring some tablets to take back into the mountains warranted my being woken. My only sanctuary was my journal. In it I recorded patients' names and operation notes, and sights beyond comprehension: massed refugees, dying babies, bodies emerging from hillsides where they'd been hastily buried. That battered notebook became the repository of my fear and guilt, that each next crisis would be the one I'd fail. But while I wrote, the people around me seemed to assume that I was doing something important – unlike sleeping or eating – and would for a brief time leave me alone.

Some pages from the journal and a couple of my photographs appeared later in a book published on the history of the Kurdish struggle, and at the book launch in a London hotel I fell into conversation with another attender at the gathering. He was a likeable, round-faced fellow in baggy tweed jacket and brogues, who might have been a professor of languages. Peering through his smudged spectacles at the caterer's choice of wines, he proposed instead a whisky at the hotel bar. There he revealed that he knew who I was; he had been on the 'intelligence side' of the aborted Kuwait rescue, responsible for putting together the operation team.

'How did you come to consider me?' I asked.

'Oh,' he said, sipping his malt, 'we'd checked up on you.'

Previously these words would have evoked a shiver of dread, but I felt less vulnerable now to their malevolent thrall. Fewer things had the power to frighten me; I had travelled too far into the realm my father had known, of medicine and the gun. On the march to their forward position the *pesh merga* fighters had required me to carry a weapon so that I would be able to add to our defensive firepower if we attracted the attention of an Iraqi helicopter. My frontline surgical work had defined harshly the limitations of my usefulness, establishing that under desperate conditions, some of my patients would die despite my best efforts. I had been under fire, seen pain and terror and atrocious wounds and, amidst the cruelty, acts of human selflessness that transcended anything of which a God might be capable. Yet out there, all the other fears that beset me – doubt about my professional commitment, my career, finding a home – vanished in the immediacy of survival; in the midst of war I'd glimpsed a sort of shelter, an elusive peace. I continued taking breaks from my hospital work to do further medical assignments with international aid organisations. Each mission would be like stepping off a precipice, from a place of order – where I questioned my suitability – into one of uncertainty and despair. There I'd rediscover that sharp lucidity, that sense of purposefulness. And each was another piece of my life wagered.

✪

My income became haphazard, so I began filing stories with those few foreign-desk editors who'd consider running a piece, read to a copy-taker over a crackling phone-line, from some doctor in an obscure place that journalists might not reach. The pay was around ten pence a word and I'd labour mightily for my sixty or eighty pounds that would help defray the rent on my low-rent flat. The pieces I wrote were not about my medical work, except in relation to general issues of aid, intervention and war's legacy of social and environmental destruction. I'd encountered a story, while working as a doctor in northern Namibia and Mozambique, concerning a South African military intelligence operation to fund the long war of destabilisation it had waged against its neighbours. In Angola the South African–backed UNITA rebel leader Jonas Savimbi had been instructed to direct his firepower at the country's wildlife. Between 1978 and 1990 the convoys and cargo flights supplying UNITA returned with the ivory and horn of perhaps a hundred thousand elephant and ten to twenty thousand rhino. The same operation was run in Mozambique, using South Africa's proxy Renamo (Mozambique National Resistance) force. Looted rhino horn and ivory was then shipped through South African government-run sanctions-busting companies to the Middle and Far East in return for strategic materials and precious foreign exchange. My investigations became newspaper articles and a television proposal, that took me back to Mozambique to work on a documentary about the slaughter of elephants in that country's South African–directed war.

The film caught the attention of Andrew, campaigns director of a leading international environmental group, who suggested we meet for dinner. I knew his strong face and quiet intensity from the evening news, exposing environmental scandals such as the case of the *Karen B,* a ship carrying European toxic waste which he'd tracked to a tiny port in Nigeria where it regularly dumped its cargo. The outcry he'd raised had forced the ship to reload its dumped consignment, and when Andrew discovered that the UK government had covertly agreed to take the waste, his public campaign prevented the vessel berthing in any British port and brought about a change to international law that forced each country generating toxic waste to be responsible for its disposal. Now Andrew had found another potential scandal, which he wished investigated. In Peninsula Malaysia a hydroelectric project was under construction, funded by the British government's international aid budget. But instead of reducing poverty and improving welfare in underdeveloped countries, here a large sum of UK taxpayers' money appeared to be paying a rather wealthy nation to build a dam – of no clear value to its people – in the middle of a jungle reserve. There was additionally the appearance that the aid funds might have been offered in order to secure an arms deal, a use expressly forbidden by the Overseas Aid Act.

Andrew pushed back his plate and continued the story. In September 1988, Malaysian Premier Dr Mahathir Mohamed had agreed with his friend Prime Minister Margaret Thatcher to sign a billion-pound arms deal to re-equip his airforce with British-made Tornado fighters. The following month, British construction consortium Balfour Beatty (a chief contributor of political funding to Thatcher's Conservative Party) and Cementation International (from which Thatcher's son Mark received fees as a consultant) were invited to submit their budget for building a dam at a site in northern Malaysia. They calculated a figure of nearly two hundred million pounds, and in November 1988 the government formally offered this sum in tied 'Aid for Trade' to Malaysia to pay for the construction. But the Overseas Development Agency (ODA) responsible for releasing the money criticised the dam as 'uneconomic'. Malaysia cancelled the Tornado deal and the aid offer lapsed.

A year later a new arms deal was under way, with Malaysia signing a four-hundred-million pound contract for Hawk fighters from British Aerospace, another company for which Mark Thatcher worked as a consultant. The dam project was also revived, bringing renewed objection from the ODA, which called the projected costs – now doubled – 'a very bad buy'. It was overruled by the Foreign Secretary and ordered to provide 234 million pounds for the dam in the largest Aid for Trade deal ever granted. Though Balfour Beatty/Cementation International had begun construction in June 1992, it was only now, a year later, that news of the project and its contentious background were becoming known. Andrew's organisation and a group called the World Development Movement were planning to publicise the material and environmental costs of the dam, but Andrew knew only that it lay on a river called the Pergau which ran through virgin jungle near the Thai border, and he asked me if I would try to find and film the site for their campaign.

I was pleased to be returning to Malaysia, whose ports and hinterland I'd visited while working as a ship's doctor in the South China Sea. My girlfriend Tina, a media studies teacher, seemed undeterred by the investigative nature of our journey or the camera that Andrew had provided: a large professional rig, rather at odds with our image as a holidaying couple. We travelled from Singapore by rail, leaving the air-conditioned Bangkok tourist express at the small junction of Gemas. On this secondary line the train consisted of old coaches with teak fittings and canvas sunblinds. We ran in the shade of rubber plantations, clattering now and then over bridges that spanned wide, slow rivers, or following raised embankments through tracts of jungle. To the west stood the dark line of the Cameron Highlands from where, during the 1948–1960 uprising called the Malayan Emergency, communist insurgents had launched attacks on planters and tin mines and laid ambush to the troop-trains carrying British reinforcements. Our train inched through damp, fern-dripping cuttings overlooked by the gun-slits of concrete police forts.

Hiring a nondescript, locally manufactured Proton in the coastal town of Kota Barahu, we drove westwards towards monsoon-shrouded hills. The road was a causeway built above swampy forest and patches of paddy, and in places we had to give way to convoys of logging trucks that took up most of its width and forced us half onto the verge. The hills were gashed with logging trails and great depots of tree-trunks were piled at the roadside, being stacked and loaded by machines with claws like crabs. On a minor road, patchily tarred, we found the Pergau, a lazy river in a valley flanked by palm-thatched villages and the small plots of *Orang-Asli* aboriginal jungle dwellers. We watched them poling by on bamboo rafts, fishing with throw nets whose edge kissed the surface in a perfect circle of foam. There was no sign of a dam.

To the west and north lay jungle-covered ranges of blue mountains, rolling to the Thai border. During the emergency, as British forces had gradually gained the upper hand, it was to these mountains that the last 'Communist Terrorists' had retreated. Some years before, a group of aging insurgents had emerged to surrender their rusted weapons. The Malaysian authorities still regarded the area as a security zone and off the main road the only traffic we encountered was blue police Land Rovers and construction machinery. We followed behind some long-loaders carrying bulldozers to a place where a new route was being carved through the jungle. Taking the turnoff at the entry boom, I charged the Proton through vales of mud and up the track until it was out of sight of the gate, pulling in behind a four-wheel-drive pickup piled with theodolites and sighting poles.

'My uncle in England told us to come and see the dam project,' I explained to the Chinese surveyor. 'He's one of the engineers.'

'Ah, Balfour Beatty, very good.' He beamed. 'Please accompany. This is service road for reservoir,' and we loaded our video equipment into the back of his truck and set off in high-range over a roadway sliced into the side of the mountain. A moraine of toppled trees and rain-gouged earth cascaded into the jungle below. Some miles on we reached the road-head near the crest of a ridge. Pneumatic drills bored the rock prior to blasting. Bulldozers were clearing more forest and the trees creaked and leaned, crashing crown-first down the slope. We could see the line of the track slashed up the next rise. I took a quick compass bearing. The area had been home to critically endangered species including elephant, tiger, tapir, and the almost extinct Sumatran rhinoceros, but now the loggers would be eyeing the road into this previously inaccessible jungle reserve and oiling their chain saws.

A site manager arrived, a big-moustached Sikh, and seeing us filming, demanded to know who we were. I tried the story of the engineer uncle in England but he was less than impressed.

'How did you get past the guard?' he wanted to know. 'Get off this site or we'll have you arrested. I'm calling security.'

Tina gave him a guileless smile, and her cutest American accent. 'Gee, I'm sorry, it's like all my fault. He told me we'd get in trouble' – pointing at me – 'but I *really* wanted to come up here because I just *love* ...' – her gesture encompassed pulverised rock and mud and the bark of flayed trees – 'nature, y'know?'

Taking my hand, she skipped me off down the track where a tipper truck was turning; we managed to get a ride down to where we'd left our car. Judging the moment, we slipped out under the entrance boom between two lorries. The guard, who appeared to have been on the lookout for us, ran after us down the roadside as we sped away.

I suspected it would be much more difficult to get onto the main dam site. Suddenly the search, to which I'd committed ourselves so light-heartedly, seemed less of a jaunt. We were discussing just how much trouble we'd be prepared to get into for Andrew's campaign when we rounded a corner on the jungle road and found ourselves at a military checkpoint. A soldier in camouflage battle dress manned a barrier of oil drums. As we stopped I noticed a flight of wooden steps up the roadside bank and a painted sign identifying the place as an army base. An officer strode out to our mud-caked car, glancing at the back seat where we'd tossed the video camera for our getaway.

'Switch off the engine,' he ordered. 'Who are you? TV?'

Tina laughed sweetly at this notion.

I produced my old vessel ID card. 'I'm a ship's doctor on holiday. The boat's being refitted in Port Kelang for a week so my girlfriend came out to join me, touring around.'

The man examined the card intently, comparing my appearance to that of the photograph, then turned it over and perused the vessel's registration details. The cooling engine ticked. I was aware of a trickle of sweat coursing down my side. When he began reading the front again I felt compelled to break the silence. 'I met some Malaysian army people three years ago on the northern Namibian border,' I said, "part of the UN transitional force, for the elections. They were stationed at a place called Ruacana.'

The man's expression changed from wariness to amazement. 'I was at Ruacana, in 1990.'

'I remember that position you had up on the bluff overlooking the dam.'

The lieutenant opened the car door. 'Welcome,' he said, waving towards the wooden steps. 'Come up for some tea.'

We followed him up the bank and through a razor-wire fence. Within the perimeter, tents were placed along gravel paths lined with whitewashed stones. Despite its well-tended look the place had a combat-ready feel; the floor of the mess tent to which the man led us had been dug a yard into the earth to reduce the risk from shell-splinters. Indicating canvas chairs, he waved away an orderly and filled some mugs from a battered urn. We sipped the warm, sugary brew while he talked nostalgically about northern Namibia: Ombalantu, Oshikuku and the International Hotel at Oshakati. The side-sheets of the tent were rolled up, giving a view over jungle and stands of verdant bamboo, and in that place those desert names seemed touched with an extraordinary exoticism.

After tea the lieutenant showed us around. Weapons emplacements were set into the ridge, sandbagged and capped by low green roofs of tin and camouflage net. Inside one a sergeant looked northwards over the jungle canopy from behind a machine gun. Pinned to the beam above each firing slit was a sketch, showing in outline the view from that vantage. Prominent features – a tall tree, a clump of bamboo – were marked with their range in metres. I wanted to ask what enemy lurked in the mountains beyond, but limited myself to a compliment on the professionalism of the position. The officer beamed, and escorted us back to our car. Tina waved at him until the base was out of sight behind the curve.

The next morning we returned to the search. The direction of the service road had indicated that the dam might be higher upstream, and eventually we found our way to the Upper Pergau. Here the river was not much more than a large stream tumbling over boulders. At the head of the valley were extensive earthworks, with machinery on the skyline. Construction company signs and a guard post marked a site road, with a barrier across it saying 'Access Closed'. We parked opposite the gate, studying the entrance over an opened map as though discussing our route. Thinking that the lack of activity might be due to the Muslim Sabbath, we were considering trying the eccentric dam-loving tourist routine when a half-dozen Land Rovers arrived, each bearing the Balfour Beatty Cementation logo and containing an expatriate family. The lead vehicle was stopped by the uniformed guard, who spoke to the driver before raising the boom to let it in. When a second cavalcade turned up we followed them to the barrier. The guard seemed puzzled by the appearance of our unassuming Proton at the tail of the line, but I called out 'Balfour Beatty' in the firmest voice I could muster and was answered by a crisp salute. A mile further we passed the Land Rovers parked at the foot of the dam wall and a group of English-accented individuals unloading picnic hampers, who stared at us as we drove by.

We followed the track as close to the top of the wall as our car would manage, then hiked to its highest point and set up our camera. The dam was being built between two shoulders of a narrow valley, out of stone quarried from the hillsides. Set into the wall's inner curve was a concrete turbine conduit, connecting, presumably, to the reservoir reached by the road-under-construction we had explored the day before. The picnic party, busily organising themselves far below us, did not look up and presently revealed themselves to be members of that expatriate sports club – encountered usually in hot corners of the world – known as the Hash House Harriers. We watched them setting off on a run through the workroads and cuttings, following a pre-marked trail and panting in the dense air of the valley bottom. Now and then their 'halloos' and the plaintive peep of a hunting horn would rise up to where we stood filming at the top of the dam wall.

Andrew supplied the footage to UK and international news networks. As campaigns director, he was on television nightly, using the images of environmental damage to belabour the Conservative government for promoting this destructive project. Andrew had an impressive before-the-camera presence, and he backed his passion with unassailable scientific argument. The dam that we'd filmed, once built, would take two years to fill, with capacity enough only to generate power for an hour or two a day at peak demand. Malaysian consumers would be paying a hundred million pounds extra for the electricity thus produced, while the construction already under way of a massive dam in Sarawak – designed to supply the entire country's power needs, plus a large surplus for export – highlighted the utter redundancy of the Pergau project.

Apart from the destruction of wildlife habitats, logging in the jungle reserve opened up by the service roads would accelerate erosion and silting, reducing the dam's effective life to considerably less than the twenty-five years claimed by its planners. The World Development Movement took the Conservative government to court for a judgement on its Foreign Secretary's decision to overrule the Overseas Development Agency head and force the payment of aid money to a country that didn't need it, for an unsound project linked apparently to an arms deal. The verdict condemned the Foreign Secretary's arrogance in appropriating £234 million of British taxpayers' money for the dam. A couple of years later, their reputation further damaged by a stream of revelations about the sale of weapons to Saddam Hussein in the run-up to the Gulf War, the Conservatives would suffer a landslide electoral defeat.

✪

'Free your mind and your arse will follow,' was the claim of some profound dope-head graffiti near my London flat (along with 'Drugs: Just Say Maybe'), but in all my dreams of travel, of involvement in the world, I had never imagined the range of options that could present themselves by letting that career steering-shudder turn into a swerve. I worked on an investigative documentary in Japan about the hunting of dolphins on an industrial scale for their meat – filming with a hidden camera on icy pre-dawn quays as the harpoon boats unloaded – and then as a doctor in an embattled enclave of Burma's Shan State, treating insurgent fighters and hill-tribe refugees caught up in a vicious Burmese government offensive. In those places the doubts that stalked my career progression were forgotten, the question of my destiny deferred. Unpredictability is seductive, and my hospital surgery work was again interrupted when a UK investigative TV programme accepted a proposal I'd written for a documentary about a British transnational company called Thor Chemicals.

Thor had been attracted to South Africa during the time of sanctions by generous tax breaks. It manufactured mercury compounds, some with military uses, and Thor's clients included Armscor, the South African government's weapons manufacturer. Mercury contamination at the plant – the British company chairman blamed sabotage by 'environmental terrorists' – had killed one worker, while others lay on hospital wards, slowly deteriorating. But international sanctions, and the human and economic costs of the wars it was waging against its neighbours, were changing attitudes in South Africa. Mandela had been released from prison and the white government was beginning to accept that it would have to relax its stranglehold on power.

Arriving back in Durban to research the film, I reviewed my toxicological studies of the symptoms of mercury poisoning. But there were elements of the case yet more disturbing, that required the revival of forensic knowledge I had last called upon during my medical student days in Cape Town when flies had buzzed against the window-screens of the police mortuary. Thor's sales director – an Englishman and trained chemical engineer, based in its Johannesburg office – had come back from a business trip to Brazil and the next evening told his wife that he was going to a meeting. Two days later his company BMW had been spotted by some black youths, parked in a downtown lot. They'd broken into it to steal the hi-fi system and been halted by a stench of putrefaction. Exhibiting a surprising civic-mindedness, they had informed the police. The trunk of the car revealed a find of such frightfulness that I'd heard that one of the officers present was later invalided from the force with a stress-induced disorder related to the trauma of the experience.

I flew up to Johannesburg to meet the senior detective working on the case. He was based in the city's Homicide Unit, a hill-top fortress of yellow brick with sliding steel gates and a gun-slit pillbox at the entrance. He showed me the crime-scene photographs. Before death, the victim's torso had been painted neatly from collar-line to waist with a glistening metallic layer. Then he'd been dismembered with a chain saw: arms cut off; transected at the thighs and hips; finally beheaded. The police pathologist believed these injuries to have been inflicted for maximum suffering, starting with those least likely to be fatal. The man had died from blood-loss after an experience whose slightest imagining nauseated me with horror. Analysis of the material on the body revealed only that it contained mercury.

The detective, a big chap with the build of a rugby forward, was a baffled man. In the old days his job had been simple. Homicide dealt with straightforward crimes in a straightforward way: suspects would be taken into the *waarheidkamer* – the truth room – and when they came out they had spilled the beans. There were allegations that the cop had been a torturer, and that an assassination attempt – a limpet mine placed under his car, which blew up when he'd got out to open the driveway gate on his way to work – was to pay him back for the sufferings of black prisoners. But perhaps his job hadn't been so simple; there were also rumours that the bomb had been a warning from State Security operatives to deter him from investigating some venture in which they were involved. A year later the detective would be accused of running a stolen car ring, pulled off all investigations and subjected to a lengthy suspension until the charges were suddenly dropped. Right now he was just trying to do his job in a changing world, where the Afrikaner Nationalist Party that had ruled South Africa since his father's day was giving way to a Mandela-led government.

In this interregnum strange undercurrents were stirring. Ghostly hit-squads – some directed by the security forces, others operating apparently autonomously – carried out massacres and assassinations. *Mossad* agents were said to be active, intent on preventing the sale of knowledge and material from South Africa's military nuclear programme, which Israel had helped set up, to unfriendly regimes in the Middle East. Organised crime, perhaps the Russian Mafia, was being blamed for an explosion of drug-dealing and extortion. The Thor director's murder might be linked to a number of other unexplained deaths of chemical engineers whom police suspected of dealing in strategic materials, specifically a mysterious compound of mercury antimony oxide known as Red Mercury, rumoured to be a component of new-generation nuclear weapons and changing hands on the international black market for large sums of money. The man's death appeared to have the hallmarks of a gruesome warning, as though he'd been involved in a deal that went wrong.

The detective allowed me glimpses at the dossiers of some of the other cases: a chemist recently returned from Singapore, invited to a meeting in a luxury Cape Town hotel suite and bludgeoned to death, a pair of scientists abducted in Port Elizabeth and found tied together and shot, and a chemical engineer in Johannesburg who'd come back from a trip to Switzerland, apparently slaughtered his whole family with kitchen knives and then gassed himself in his company car, leaving an enigmatic note that referred to something he'd become involved in whose consequences were too severe to live with. A South African journalist who'd been working on the nuclear materials story suggested that I call a man named Stoffberg, a reputed arms trafficker. Stoffberg took my number and said he would call me back. An hour later he did. He claimed to have heard that Red Mercury was behind the deaths, including that of the Thor director, and that there was a dealer near Pretoria who had a sample of the stuff.

I thought it unwise to follow up this lead. The journalist, who often used sub-legal channels in Johannesburg for information, assured me that he could guarantee our safety. He put out the word that we represented a European buyer interested in Red Mercury. Someone called him and a meeting was arranged. I came along as a 'scientific advisor' – I had read everything I could find on the attributes of this possibly mythical compound, so that I could talk about it convincingly – and we were accompanied by 'security', a big man with a gun under his jacket. My briefcase contained some technical manuals and a notebook. It also carried a small video camera built into the base that filmed through a concealed aperture, to record what we found.

We arrived at the meeting-place some twenty miles outside Pretoria. The house was screened by gum-trees; no neighbours could see within. We walked up the path, my video camera running silently. A man who looked like a retired boxer let us in and made a phone call while we sat in a front room decorated with tapestries of cats. A few minutes later a Mercedes with tinted windows rolled up the driveway. I hoped we'd brought enough protection. The dealers – a paunchy fellow in a suit and a nervous man with greased-back hair – smoked a couple of cigarettes each while they made small talk in heavy Afrikaner accents. Then they produced from under the bath a metal canister and took the top off.

'Looks like unrefined yellow-cake uranium,' I said. 'We're not interested.'

'Just checking, hey,' they sniffed, lighting up again while the boxer went outside and came back with a couple of heavy sealed bottles of a shiny red-grey sludge which he put down in front of me on the coffee table. The contents resembled the descriptions of Red Mercury I'd read, and authentic-looking laboratory assay labels on the bottles identified the contents as mercury antimony oxide. I made a show of comparing the assay specifications to my technical manual while the hidden camera rolled and my colleague chatted to the men. They were anxious for a deal.

'We scheme to retire from this business,' said the Brylcreemed one, 'so you can tell your buyer we'll take any reasonable offer.'

Some of the covert footage ended up being used in the Thor Chemicals documentary, but that film was more about corporate responsibility by a UK parent company and lack of worker protection in South Africa. Once it had been edited and transmitted, the TV commissioning editor asked me to return to South Africa to follow the Red Mercury story. I revisited my acquaintance at the Johannesburg Homicide Unit. He was sitting glumly in his office behind the fortified walls. A newspaper article on the desk in front of him discussed the police's failure to make any headway in their investigation of the Red Mercury killings. Over a picture of the detective and two of his blocky colleagues was a headline that read 'Gorillas in the Mist'.

'I'm sick of this shit,' he said. 'Me and my men has too much to do as it is. Everyone's shooting each other. We catch them and takes them to court but the legal system's back-logged, so they gets bail. The next day the cunts is on the phone, saying they going to kill us. I got officers on sick leave, taking early retirement, the whole force is falling apart. And these fucking deaths doesn't stop.' Stoffberg had been found dead with his wife, having apparently shot her before putting the gun to his own head. Another arms dealer – an alleged associate of the murdered Thor director – appeared to have killed himself by the unusual expedient of tying over his head a plastic bag from which a tube ran to a cylinder of cyanide gas. The detective rubbed his lumpy face.

'Come and have a *dop*,' he said, and we went upstairs to a small bar in the police station where cabinets of pistol trophies lined the wall. A couple of cops were whacking darts into a board suspended beneath a set of kudu horns. The detective introduced the other officers to me as fellow members of the Red Mercury investigating team. They shook my hand and chewed on their mouthfuls of beer, and everyone nodded into their drinks and admitted that they were making *vok-all* progress and that I might as well be given access to the material if I wanted.

For the next week I sat in an office, ploughing through autopsy reports and the glossy prints of the police photographers. They documented lethal and defensive wounds, bloody footprints, the shocked faces of the violently dead. A sergeant brought me coffee and a selection of plastic bags from the evidence room: blood-clotted knives, a German automatic with hair on the front sight, a broken wristwatch. I pored over photocopies of the dead men's passports detailing their movements, and their desk diaries that listed meetings with other victims. The scientists might simply have known each other through being in a shared field of work – perhaps they and the arms dealers also had legitimate business links – but those who knew the answers were dead or keeping just as quiet.

In the world of fiction, of course, I would have tied together the murders by skilful sleuthing, proved the involvement of the security services or *Mossad* or nuclear black-marketeers and solved the case, but this was South Africa, where conspiracy flourished and people died all the time in abrupt ways. Driving around Johannesburg to examine suburban homes, freshly repainted, that had been recent death scenes, or flying down to Cape Town and Durban to talk to potential witnesses, I began to be troubled by increasing paranoia. A thief whose arm I grabbed as he reached through my car window in an attempt to snatch my briefcase addressed me as 'Doctor'. Before climbing into my vehicle I'd spend ten minutes looking around and under it, trying to spot the explosive package that was waiting to blow me away. I sent back daily reports in code to the television company's Manchester headquarters, but the link between the deaths remained stubbornly circumstantial. I was relieved when eventually the commissioning editor decided that the project was unfilmable and called me back to London.

❖

I kept intending to settle back into my professional career – to be a full-time hospital surgeon, stay in one place and make a worthwhile contribution to society – but my work amidst repression and pillage and random death had stolen from me some belief in the endurability of human endeavour. I had hoped that being back in South Africa would offer some fulfilment. Instead I'd felt estranged, as though I could never again trust the easy assurance of having a place I knew as home. My past in that country was being erased: crazy Graeme the scientist, in a suicide pact with his partner that involved champagne, cocaine and the exhaust of his Mercedes directed into the bedroom of their Johannesburg home; the body of my gypsy ex-lover Linda found in a mystery car-crash eight hundred miles from Cape Town, a corpse beside her that was not that of her husband. My close childhood friend, blond Greg the Boer, had joined the air force, tried flying and ended up a game warden on a wildlife reserve outside Durban. He'd been stalking thieves who used the reserve as a contraband route, when they got the drop on him and fired first and he bled to death on the veld. It seemed to me better to die for something than for nothing, and I considered the proposals of various medical intervention organisations for war surgery assignments in dangerous places like Sri Lanka and Sarajevo and Chechnya.

My friend Andrew's life was undergoing its own vicissitudes. The environmental organisation to which he'd given his energies for the past ten years was changing. Its new director eschewed Andrew's style of issue-driven campaigning as too confrontational. He favoured instead the idea of a participatory relationship with government and industry, possibly because of his closer affinity to the Establishment than to the disrespectful, dedicated activists who made environmental groups so effective. But Andrew had a plan for our mutual salvation: we would work together on our own independent film project. He was convinced that with my experience of making investigative documentaries and his expertise in environmental issue-raising, we'd be able to put together a proposal for a conservation documentary irresistible to any commissioning editor. His aim – to try to pre-empt the destruction of a rare, untouched bit of the planet – offered the chance for redemption my life rather desperately needed.

Andrew had discovered that Rio Tinto Zinc (RTZ), the global mining transnational, was expecting to get World Bank funding and an agreement from the Malagasy government to start mining along Madagascar's southern coast, with incalculable environmental and social consequences. UK-based RTZ had a history of projects around the world – Canada, Australia, Sierra Leone – that had brought conflict with indigenous people. In the Pacific, their vast mine on Bougainville provoked protest from the islanders about their land being stolen; the answering repression from security forces, which RTZ was accused of sanctioning, had sparked an armed rebellion. The company's Madagascar plan was to repeat an operation they'd been running for a decade in South Africa, strip-mining coastal sand dunes for titanium dioxide. The mineral – found as glinting black granules in beach sand – is refined into a whitener for makeup, mayonnaise and toothpaste. I'd seen their South African mine while working at a hospital in Zululand. Coastal dunes had been bulldozed into a vast hollow, which was then flooded to create an artificial lake. On it, a floating line of tall dredgers advanced night and day, scooping sand from the front edge of the lake, centrifuging it to extract the minerals and then dumping it from their sterns to back-fill the lake behind them. Bulldozers worked ahead of the dredgers, clearing dune forest that had existed for millennia; behind stretched a desert of scoured beach-sand for the wind to lift and blow away.

South Africa conservationists had thwarted RTZ's attempt to expand its operation to the nearby St Lucia marine reserve – its wetlands a World Heritage site – and the corporation was looking at new sources of titanium dioxide. Impoverished Madagascar had hardly any conservation movement, despite its evolutionary uniqueness. Its lemurs and eighty-five percent of its plants are exclusive to the island, along with ninety-eight percent of the reptiles and half of its birds and bats. Andrew discovered that the Environmental Impact Assessment of the mining area which RTZ had been required to commission had revealed sixteen types of plants previously unknown, with one part of the intended extraction site showing 'the highest diversity of reptile life recorded anywhere in Madagascar'. The dredgers would hoover up fifty miles of mangrove, lagoons and dune forest, displacing coastal villagers who would lose their homes and ancestral burial grounds. This was the catastrophe we hoped to prevent.

The steps between submitting a documentary proposal and seeing it commissioned can take up to a year. We had to work much faster than that if we were to challenge RTZ's Madagascar plans before environmental destruction began. Andrew's ardour and excitement swept me on. Over meals with him and his partner Chris at their London flat, we spread our maps on the dinner table and set to work framing the proposal. I made provisional approaches to commissioning editors that I'd worked with previously, but those who returned my calls all wanted to see footage before they would talk further. Andrew and I decided to spend December on an unobtrusive four-week filming reconnaissance of the island's southern coast – we did not want to attract attention from the mining company or the Malagasy authorities prematurely – arriving back in London at the start of the new year to edit our material into a visual proposal. RTZ was expected to receive its funding for the operation in February 1995, by which time we hoped to have our documentary commissioned in order to start formal filming by April. Some months before our planned departure Andrew had introduced the entomologist into the project.

'He's got amazing knowledge of Madagascar wildlife,' he enthused. 'He'll be a real asset.'

I saw the man's insect photographs, with their lapidary eyes. It was true that he seemed informed and motivated, though rather remote; my yardstick for choosing a travelling companion, especially in places where one might run foul of officialdom, was whether I could face spending time in a police cell in their company. I comforted myself with the thought of Andrew's warm humour, and we began our preparations for the trip.

My role, as well as investigative, would be to share the filming, and I helped Andrew choose a compact professional video camera, tripod and audio rig. Also, my previous travels in Madagascar helped to prepare for the range of risks the place could offer. Some roads were unsafe because of armed bandits. People travelled along the coast in big outrigger sailing canoes; I'd been in one that was been blown out of sight of land by a sudden storm that ripped away our sail and began to shake lose the bindings that kept the craft together. I had expected to drown, though I revised our likely cause of death subsequently when I inspected the shark-bite ward at the local hospital. The case that impressed me most was a man who had been perched on the gunwale of his canoe – a good yard above the water – when a rampaging shark had launched itself from the depths like a torpedo to remove his buttock with one slashing bite. Such dangers could not be guarded against, only avoided, but I hoped at least to prevent us becoming ill. When I'd fallen sick with bacillary dysentery, the students with whom I was staying in the capital Antananarivo had managed to obtain a forged prescription for the necessary medication – a valuable therapeutic skill if one was near a pharmacy, but less useful in the wilds of southern Madagascar. Besides filming, I would also be the expedition doctor. I packed antibiotics, treatment for diarrhoeal illnesses and oral rehydration mixture, intravenous fluid and infusion sets: an emergency survival kit. My experiences in travel and film-making and medicine and my friendship with Andrew, all brought together, seemed to have made me for this venture.

7

Natural Causes

The voice on the phone belonged to Chris, Andrew's partner. She sounded distraught.

'I've been at the airport all day,' she said. 'Andrew was supposed to fly back from Madagascar to Paris overnight and then on to London this morning. I thought maybe he'd missed his connection, so I waited and waited. I'm so worried.'

A cramp of concern and guilt gripped my chest, for – after almost a year of research and planning – I hadn't been with Andrew on the trip. As the time had neared for our departure I was dealing with a medical crisis closer to home.

A doctor friend whom I'd known since South Africa, where we'd been colleagues together, had suffered a setback with his drug problem. Caught injecting at a London hospital, he'd gone on the run and sent me a plea for help. I persuaded him to return home and went to meet him at his apartment. His breath smelt cold and chalky, and he cried and shook. I took him to a hospital, where he was entered into a drug dependency programme. Then I contacted the UK Medical Council, explaining that my friend had voluntarily submitted himself for treatment, and asked them not to start disciplinary proceedings that might have him struck off the practitioners' register. Between his outpatient sessions it was essential that he should not be alone and so I moved in with him. Searches of the cupboards revealed ampoules of drugs, which I destroyed. I tried to limit his drinking – in his despair he was swallowing a bottle of vodka a day – and to encourage him to take solid food; we would sit through laborious meals where he'd chew and gag, unable to swallow. With the Madagascar departure date fast approaching, I told Andrew, regretfully, that I'd be unable to accompany him and explained the reasons; I promised that we'd start editing the footage into a proposal as soon as he got back, and assured him of my presence on the return trip in April.

The night before Andrew's departure I had visited him at his flat for a final equipment check. He and Chris and I opened a bottle of wine and drank to good fortune, and planned a shot-list of ideal, felicitous images. Through his excitement at going to Madagascar – environmentalist's heaven – it was clear that Andrew was worried. His differences with his organisation's director had culminated in a long fax received that day, delineating the end of his employment with the group and discussing the conditions of his severance. Environmental film-making was now more than just a venture; Andrew was depending on it to provide his future career. Anxiety filled me at the weight of his expectations and I wished painfully that I could be going with him. I crossed my fingers that the reconnaissance trip would be successful.

The postcards that I'd received from him suggested that it was. Andrew described his intense schedule – tramping through mangrove and jungle, staying in village huts, up before dawn to catch the first light – full of a true delight at the diversity of this paradise. But there was sadness too at being far from home for Christmas and New Year and I knew that – no matter how perfectly the filming was going – he would not voluntarily have missed his return flight.

'Did you see the entomologist at the airport?' I asked Chris. 'He and Andrew were supposed to be travelling back together.'

'No, I didn't, though I looked for him. Then I decided I'd somehow missed Andrew too, and dashed home, but when I got back the flat was empty. I called the entomologist and he said that Andrew had probably got lost for a day in the forest and missed his flight and that he'd turn up any moment, but I've got this terrible feeling that something bad has happened. I want to go to Madagascar and find him. I'd like you to come with me.'

'Of course I will,' I said. 'Let's see what we can find out from the entomologist in the meantime.'

'He's asleep,' said the man's girlfriend when I phoned to say that Chris and I were coming over. 'He's had a long flight and he's very tired,' and indeed the entomologist seemed somewhat put out at our arrival. He explained that he had seen Andrew setting off, on the afternoon of the last day in December, to do some final filming at a place called Petriky Forest, fifteen miles along the coast from the town of Fort Dauphin where they were staying. He'd noticed Andrew's absence at the hotel New Year's Eve party that night, and that Andrew had not returned by the next morning. Leaving instructions to organise a search, the entomologist had flown back to the capital Antananarivo for his scheduled flight to Paris, his intention, he explained, being to bring the news back to London.

I asked him if he knew what might have happened to Andrew. The man's reply carried a note of exasperation.

'Andrew was difficult to work with; really stubborn. He was always blundering about, chatting to people in his non-existent French. We ended up working apart, so that's why I wasn't with him on that last visit to Petriky. I've no idea where he got to. Maybe he wandered off into the forest, met some villager and got speared for the money in that belly-bag he wore. The camera alone would have been worth more than a Malagasy peasant could earn in his entire life.'

Chris, beside me, took a tremulous breath. Hoping to forestall further tactlessness, I took out a notepad and asked the entomologist to draw a map of the area where Andrew had gone. He sketched a bay with a lagoon separated from the sea by a bar, a line of inland hills – high dunes, covered by bush – and between these features the expanse of Petriky Forest extending along the coast. I asked for more details, about villages and roads.

'I think you're making too much of this,' the man objected. 'I mean, all he has to do is head south and he'll hit the sea, or north and he'll be on the hills. He's probably back at the hotel already, planning to get on the next flight.'

'There's no phone link to Fort Dauphin,' said Chris, 'but I've just spoken to the British ambassador in Antananarivo and he's in radio communication with the Fort Dauphin gendarmes and there's no sign of Andrew. He was last seen on Saturday afternoon. Now it's Monday midnight over there, so he's been gone around two and a half days. Jonathan and I are leaving in the morning to go and look for him.'

A disconcerted look crossed the entomologist's face. 'Shit,' he muttered. 'Maybe I should have stayed.'

I packed in a hurry: lightweight clothing, jungle boots, a hat and a bush-jacket, plus an English-French dictionary to back up my half-remembered Malagasy French. I included a medical resuscitation kit and drugs for the treatment of infections prevalent in the region, including malaria and dengue fever. Finally, in case Andrew had been injured, I added the compact set of surgical instruments I carried when working as a war surgeon.

Chris spoke little on the long flight from London via Paris to the Malagasy capital. From there our plane flew south over jungled mountains, to circle above the small town of Fort Dauphin on its peninsula, edged by bluffs and headlands and white beaches. Some two- and three-story concrete buildings marked the main street, but much of the town consisted of palm-thatch roofs along dirt roads, interspersed with casuarina trees and coco-palms. Wrecked cargo ships, beached by old storms, rusted outside the harbour break-water. We dropped low over a placid lagoon and trundled to a halt on the landing strip. Waiting for us was the tall, pony-tailed figure of Mark, an American conservationist based in the town, who had helped Andrew with his research and been among the first people to make a search of the area where he'd gone missing.

As he drove us into town, Mark outlined the events around Andrew's disappearance. On the Saturday afternoon Andrew had engaged a driver – the same man who'd taken him to Petriky on previous visits – and travelled to the hills overlooking the forest. He'd filmed from the top, then set off down the slope, saying he'd be back before sunset. At dusk the driver had begun to blow his horn. When Andrew had failed to appear after a couple of hours he'd gone back to town to inform the vehicle-hire owner, then returned to the hilltop. There he spent the night, hooting and flashing his headlights. The next morning the driver had accompanied some local police to visit villages on the forest edge and question the inhabitants, to no avail. Mark and the commander of the district's gendarme unit mounted a search the following day, mobilising men from the settlement nearest to where Andrew had entered the forest, and the day before our arrival the police had again visited the villages. So far, no trace of Andrew had been found.

The *gérant d'hotel* – the manager – greeted Chris and I with gentle solicitude. He had helped organise the search and, after making a detailed list of Andrew's possessions for the *commissaire de police,* had sealed his room pending instructions. The man showed us through an inner courtyard to rooms that overlooked the harbour. He paused at my door to speak to me. Andrew had been *'un gentilhomme, toujours calme,'* he told me. He'd seen him leave that last afternoon for the forest, *impeccable* as always, though he understood that Andrew had been suffering a stomach illness for the previous few days.

Mark walked us down the main street to police headquarters, an old French colonial building painted in a flaking yellow wash. Goats grazed around the compound's entrance and Morse code squeaked from under the tiled eaves of the veranda. In the gloom of his office the crisply uniformed *commissaire de police* stood up from behind his desk – a separate chair bore his silver-braided blue kepi – and shook our hands. Then he opened a dossier and began to read aloud. The first page stated his authority as head of the investigation. The second summarised what had been established: On the afternoon of the last day of the last year, *le disparu* – the disappeared – took a car to Petriky. There he left the car and went into the forest. He was seen again by no-one. The *commissaire* turned to the driver's statement, which he read in the first person, giving the man's words an affecting emphasis: 'Night falls. I call, I sound the horn. Nothing. The darkness is profound. I wait and wait...'

All the *commissaire*'s researches had proved fruitless. There had been no information from the villagers; an accident or injury remained a possibility. He talked about the *charbonniers du bois,* the charcoal-makers, who fell trees in the middle of the forest and set the wood slow-burning in a deep pit covered by sand. 'Perhaps your friend has fallen in such a pit,' he ventured. A gendarmerie dog team was on standby at the capital to fly in to Fort Dauphin to participate in the search, and a helicopter could also be obtained. It was up to us to authorise such steps, for their cost would have to be met from outside sources. Chris had already discussed such options with the British ambassador; we requested that the dog team be sent for right away.

My friendship with Andrew had grown from my work for him as an investigator. Now, in Fort Dauphin, I was trying to discover what could have happened to him. I explored the matter of Andrew's illness, mentioned by the *gérant*. Mark hadn't known that Andrew was unwell. He'd heard from an American Peace Corps volunteer running a nursery in a distant village that Andrew had visited him, found him sick with dysentery and handed over the necessary medication, presumably from the treatment kit I'd organised.

There was the question of local feelings regarding the mine and whether Andrew's research might have raised the ire of someone sufficiently to do him in. Mark believed this was improbable. Andrew, discussing his research and the filming he'd done, had made no mention of any hostility. Most of the fishermen and villagers who lived along the stretch of coast threatened by the mining had known nothing of the project until Andrew asked them about it. Even those in the town who might be expecting to be made rich by the mine would have been unlikely to have taken action against a visiting naturalist, which is how Andrew had represented himself.

I asked Mark his opinion of the entomologist's suggestion that Andrew had been speared in the bush by a tribesman for his video camera. Mark discounted it. The Antandry, though deadly hunters, lived by bartering meat for what they needed from other tribes; a villager walking into town to sell a camera to one of the Asian shopkeepers – the only way to convert it into cash – would have roused acute suspicion.

That afternoon Andrew's driver took me to the forest. The road ran westwards along the coast between mountains and lakes. Now and then it crossed a river on a clattering box-girder bridge, where we'd have to wait while herds of wide-horned zebu picked their way over the metal roadway. Desirée was a man in his sixties, chosen by Andrew because he was steady in his work. He talked about the journeys they'd made together around the region. On his arm was a wristwatch that Andrew had given him as a Christmas present.

'He will return in April,' Desirée said. 'That is what he told me.'

We left the road at a place marked by tyre-tracks turning off into the bush, and bumped over rough ground until a trail appeared. After some miles of careful driving, Desirée pulled up on the brow of a hill. A steady wind off the sea ruffled the forest below. It glowed in the afternoon light, a dense cover of green pinched at this point to a couple of miles' width between the hill and the lagoon. East and west it filled the coastal plain, and in the distance a village could be seen, hemmed by a checkerboard of bright rice fields.

'This is where he walked,' said Desirée, pointing down the hillside, 'with his brown camera bag and his other long *sac* on his shoulder.'

'I'm going to take a look down there.'

Desirée said nothing, staring at the trees below.

'I will be back in under one hour,' I assured him. We compared the time on our watches. 'If you do not see me by then, start sounding the horn.'

As I descended, the forest began to take on detail. Tall trees stuck above the canopy, their leaves a pale green. Others were almost red, or of variegated green and gold. At the forest edge I tried to see within but the foliage formed a dense screen. Taking a last glance up to where I'd left Desirée, I ducked my head and stepped through the wall of leaves.

I suppose I'd imagined all along that Andrew was alive; hurt, perhaps, but surviving on rainwater and boiled sweets, or limping through the undergrowth on some desperate trek. Now my hopes faded. There was nothing in this place that could sustain life. The wind I'd felt up on the hill, that swayed the tree-tops, did not reach here and the air was hot and stale. Dry leaf-dust coated my face as I pushed deeper into the forest. The dune-sand underfoot was exhausting to trudge through. Lianas snared my ankles and thorns lashed themselves around my body, arresting my progress. Layers of canopy above cut off all view of the sky. It was almost impossible to see more than a yard or so, for head-height foliage made it necessary to stoop and thick undergrowth obscured the ground; I realised that Andrew could be lying a few feet away, entirely invisible. After forty minutes I stumbled onto a tiny track that led me back to the hill's foot. It was clear that a proper search would need large numbers of men, and that a helicopter might prove useless.

That evening the *gérant,* having received authorisation from the police, opened Andrew's room. It was as he'd left it before setting off that last afternoon: bag half packed on the bed, notes and gifts packaged, a pair of Antandry tribal spears leaning in a corner awaiting wrapping, their forged points sharp as needles.

Chris glanced at them and shuddered. 'Take those away, please,' she said.

We'd begun the disturbing process of sorting though Andrew's possessions when Mark arrived, accompanied by a man in green battle dress with a strong, high-cheekboned face.

'This is the *commandant du brigade* of the gendarmes,' he said, 'the person who's been conducting the searches.'

'*Monsieur le Médecin,*' said Commandant Jean formally, shaking my hand. He bowed to Chris and apologised for his failure to find the fiancé of Mademoiselle. From a box he produced the video-tapes secured from Andrew's luggage, which he wished to view with us in case they contained clues. Mark had brought a camera and monitor on which we watched the footage, Mark identifying the lagoons and forests while the commandant summarised the comments of farmers in paddy fields, fishermen repairing nets and elders at the doors of their huts, learning that their villages and livelihoods lay in the path of the extractor dredgers.

'It seems that many already know M'sieur Andrew,' said Jean. 'We will need their assistance in our search. It has rained in the forest and the dogs may have difficulty finding his trail.'

The next morning, with the dog team en route from the capital, we accompanied Commandant Jean and a detachment of his men to recruit a search-party. The few villages in Petriky were inaccessible by road and we parked the trucks and walked for hours along the forest edge. On the outskirts of each settlement we'd wait while the commandant went to request an audience with the headman. Visible through the trees would be the sacred grove of the village burial ground, with its palisade of poles carrying impaled zebu skulls like horned totems. These sacrifices to the spirits of the dead were the only sign of surplus in the palm-thatch hamlets. In the shade, grass mats would be laid on which we sat before the elders, the rest of the village ranged in a circle around us. Each meeting started with a request for the assistance of the ancestors. The village *sorcier* would pour a libation of rum against a tree-trunk; in the heat it evaporated immediately, filling the air with a smell of caramel.

Chris passed round some pictures of Andrew, to comments and exclamations; it was clear that the villagers recognised Andrew from his wanderings through the area. The elders debated his possible location, the number of men that could be spared to comb the forest and how much they'd receive for their time. We had discussed this vital issue in advance with Commandant Jean, for villagers had lost work-days in previous searches, while the Antanouche villagers, unlike the hunters of the Antandry, were farmers and fishermen who preferred not to venture far into the forest. Some believed it to be the abode of a malevolent spirit called *Pakafou* – the Stealer of Hearts – that could take possession of a man and cause his body to vanish, and suspected this might have been Andrew's fate. An additional incentive was announced, in the form of a reward of one million francs Malagasy payable to whomever found Andrew, and I carried in my backpack, along with my resuscitation kit, some rubber-band-bound blocks of banknotes to meet these expenses.

Well before dawn the next morning we loaded ourselves, Commandant Jean's unit and the now-arrived dog team into the trucks we'd hired. The first light had just touched the tops of the forest when we parked at the hilltop. On the slope below were gathered perhaps two hundred men in ragged shorts and palm-leaf hats, carrying spears or axes or rice sickles, each with the broad, cracked feet of someone who has never worn shoes. First the dog-team went down to the forest, where the animals were given the scent from Andrew's clothes. The gendarmes from the capital wore camouflage uniform and held themselves a little aloof from their rural colleagues; their poise didn't survive the moment when the dogs bounded off into the dense growth, yelping with excitement, dragging their handlers behind them as they quartered the ground for a trail. Commandant Jean followed, with Chris and I. The sun was yet low but the air in the forest was already stifling. Men and dogs panted, wet with sweat. After half an hour the dog crews were withdrawn to check the next sector. Chris went with them. The men, who had been sitting quietly in their village groups, rose to their feet and formed up along the forest edge.

We stood shoulder to shoulder, gendarmes spaced at intervals along the line. Commandant Jean had issued orders to his men that all weapons must be on safety, and only fired – two shots in the air – if a significant find was made. Then, at a shout from the commandant, we plunged into the green shadow. For a short time I could see the men beside me, for a while longer hear their crackling, tearing progress. Then only an occasional voice sounded, far away, and the dull chop of machetes. I thumped my stick against the tree-trunks but the noise was swallowed up. Curtains of thorn hung me up for minutes at a time; as I unhooked one strand, more would twine themselves around me, or try to claw the rucksack from my back. It was impossible to proceed in a straight line. I cursed my incompetence at packing so fast in London that I'd forgotten to bring a compass. The four litres of water I was carrying were revealed as utterly inadequate in the steam-bath heat, for whatever I drank left my pores at once in a flood of sweat, without alleviating my brick-dry throat.

For an unknown time, I realised, I had heard no calls, no distant axe-blows. Remembering the entomologist's suggestion of Andrew falling victim to a jungle spear, I was seized by dread; if he was right, then the perpetrator would probably be here in the forest with me, another blundering Westerner with a bag full of money. In a claustrophobic panic I charged forward, but at once the thorns seized me in their elastic embrace and I tore myself free only at the cost of a trouser-leg ripped down the seam. Then the ground collapsed and I found myself chest-deep in an old *charbonnier*'s pit, trying to kick my way out through carbonised branches that crumbled under my boots. Looking up for a handhold, I was suddenly transfixed by a sight that calmed my breathless fear: the rich blue sky, seen though the gap in the canopy where the *charbonnier* had felled the tree to make his charcoal. Around the edges of the gap, leaves flexed in the prevailing wind, and I knew now in which direction lay the sea.

I came out at the edge of the lagoon and sank down in the shade. Here and there, scattered along its shoreline, sat other men. We waved. More stragglers emerged, including the gendarmes. Commandant Jean was among the last to appear and he looked like the rest of us: sweat-slathered, dusty, his face and arms stitched with thorn-scratches. He held a conference. No-one had found a trace of Andrew's passage. Our spirits low, we filed back along a forest path that led to our starting point on the hillside. The drivers had fetched rations in the form of cooked yams, which were piled on tarpaulins, and the tired men tucked themselves into the skirts of bushes out of the hard sunlight and began to eat. They spoke together in low voices, exclaiming only when a snake wound its way through one of the groups.

I was sitting with Chris in the shade when a gendarme approached, saying that the Commandant requested my presence to confer about the next sector of the search. As we were studying the map the sergeant appeared and spoke in his superior's ear. Commandant Jean listened, his face still. Then he relayed the news: during the meal-break one of the villagers had reportedly spotted a *tengray*, a sort of edible rodent. Chasing it along the forest edge, he'd wounded the animal with a machete-throw, whereupon it had dived into the forest. Pursuing it deep under the trees, however, he'd encountered *une sensation mauvaise* – the hunter's words were difficult to translate – and wished to take us to the place. I went back and told Chris that one of the searchers thought there was an area where we should look. Her face suffused at once with hope, but I suggested gently that she wait for me to return with information about whether there was any significance to the man's tale. I saw her glance at my backpack medical kit and I picked it up. Then Jean and I and the sergeant walked down to where our guide waited. Behind us, a silence had fallen on the watching crowd.

The hunter was a small, sharp-faced man whom I realised I had noticed before. At our visit the previous day to his village he'd sat silently, listening to the request for searchers – I wasn't sure if anything had distinguished him apart from a certain watchfulness – and today I'd been aware of his gaze as we'd straggled back from the rendezvous at the lagoon. He acknowledged my approach with the briefest of nods before taking up his machete and setting off in a rapid walk along the forest edge. Commandant Jean gazed after the man with a speculative look. Then, accompanied by the sergeant and another gendarme, we set off behind our guide. After walking for around twenty minutes – a longer distance, somehow, than seemed consistent with the hunter's account – we turned into the forest. No trail was apparent and we followed the man in single file, bent almost double as he chopped a low path with his machete.

After a time we found ourselves scrambling up the branches of a downed tree. In falling it had crushed its neighbours, opening a long gap in the canopy. We walked along the trunk, which formed a bridge above the surrounding foliage. A smell came to meet us, that I'd first encountered in that blown-up tank in the Sinai; not sickly-sweet like those who've never known it say, but sour and unbanishable, like human sweat a thousand times concentrated, or the acid reek that tarnished brass leaves on the fingertips. At the tree's end, where the roots had been torn from the ground, we looked down on a small clearing not much longer than a man.

Andrew lay face down, his length outstretched as if he'd dived from the sky; indeed, it appeared almost that the foliage had been sundered by his fall, for though it stood dense and high about, the lianas formed a dip around him as though subsided under some great weight. His head was towards us, crown exposed to the sun, showing the bald spot he had always managed to hide. Despite the foreshortening of our vantage point he looked immensely tall, his body spanning a distance much greater that it could have encompassed in life.

Jean prevented us from jumping down while he studied the scene. Ashes from an old fire lay across the clearing, stippled with the marks of raindrops. No tracks were visible apart from those of insects and small paws. We descended and approached the body. Andrew's face lay against a khaki-coloured camera bag. His hands were raised, fingers locked in the straps of the bag on either side as though he might have been trying to use it to pull himself upright as he died.

'Peut-être pour protéger la tête,' Jean suggested, lifting his arms as though to shield his face from a blow. Plucking a twig, he indicated a matted crust on the back of Andrew's neck. Then he hooked back the collar, revealing a cleft in the livid skin: *'Coup de machete?'*

I suspected that the skin had split under pressure from the cloth-edge, for it was evident that Andrew had been dead for days in the tropical heat. Deliquescence was well advanced, so that his hair and clothes and skin shone as though soaked in oil, impregnating the cloth of the tripod case, which was still slung over one shoulder – suggesting that his end had been quick – and the canvas belt of the belly-bag around his waist. Only his brogues, their leather dusted with the ash of the clearing, were dry. The soles pointed skyward and as I looked at the heels, worn away on London pavements, I felt my heart slow like the tolling of a dirge. Grief, dull and heavy, settled on my shoulders.

Leaving the sergeant on guard – he moved upwind, lighting a cigarette of rough black tobacco – we cut our way back to open ground. Outside the forest I hawked and spat but the smell lay in the back of my throat, tainting each breath. Jean left the other gendarme to wait at the place where we'd emerged, to guide the officers who would be sent back to secure the site. Then we set off back towards the gathering that waited for us at the foot of the hill.

'He speaks no French,' said Jean, indicating our guide, who walked a few paces ahead. *'Alors,* what do you think?'

'Andrew's clothes did not appear disturbed, or his pockets.' I knew that soon I would have to speak to Chris, at that moment still waiting hopefully for news, and I concentrated on my reply. 'The camera bag was closed and the money bag he wore on his waist was still there. I do not think the body was moved after death. But the man who took us there, I think he knew that the body was there all along.'

Jean nodded. 'Perhaps he was frightened to say before, frightened of being arrested. And then he became worried that *le disparu* might be found by someone else and he would lose the reward.' The subject of our conversation glanced back as we spoke and I sensed his fear: at being blamed for the white man's death, of losing everything.

'We will take him back to the town with us,' said Jean. 'He will come readily, for he wants the money. We will bring back the body of your friend and see if we can discover what killed him.'

We came in sight of the waiting men, and again silence fell. Then, perhaps reading our mood, a murmur grew and swelled across the slope. I walked straight towards where Chris sat. She smiled as she saw me but I was unable to respond, and at once her face became pale and set. I knelt beside her.

'Chris, I'm so sorry.'

She said nothing, her head down, twining her fingers in her lap.

'I think he died quickly, on that day he went into the forest. I don't think he suffered.'

She asked if she could see him. I thought of Andrew's body dissolving into the sand, his fingers clawing the camera bag in that futile gesture of resurrection, and the miasma of decay that filled the clearing.

'Perhaps it would be better to wait until he's been brought back to town.'

Chris allowed me to lead her through the throng of villagers. The men held to their chests their battered hats. At the car Desirée opened the door for her, in his eyes such a soft compassion that I felt tears start. Chris looked straight ahead. I wished I could indicate that I shared her grief, and touched her shoulder as we drove back to town through the light of that sad afternoon. Back at the hotel she said nothing apart from asking me if I had some medication that would help her sleep.

I looked through my treatment kit, but this was not a situation I had provided for, so I sought out Desirée and asked if he could drive me to the town's hospital. It was a small place of perhaps forty beds, in design like other tropical hospitals I'd seen in Africa and Asia. The physician on duty was a short, Chinese-looking man with spectacles thick as bottle-bottoms. I began explaining my presence in Fort Dauphin, but he seemed already to know who I was.

'I am sorry for your loss, *Docteur*,' he said as he opened the pharmacy and gave me some sedatives. 'Let me know if there is more I can do.'

The next morning I found the gendarmerie sergeant waiting; Commandant Jean had requested that *Monsieur le Médicin* might assist the police doctor with the examination of the deceased, who had been brought into the town during the night. I asked who had carried out this grim task and learned that a score of villagers had cleared a track by torchlight through the bush to reach the body, which – under the direction of the commandant and the town's undertaker – they'd doused in rum to try to suppress the smell. Then they'd borne it on a stretcher out of the forest and up the hill to a waiting truck.

The sergeant led me through the police compound to a low concrete room, set among bushes near the perimeter fence. A man in a red rubber apron stood outside, smoking a cigarette. He raised a hand as I approached.

'*Bonjour, Docteur,*' he called, and I recognised the Chinese-looking physician from the hospital. Piled beside the building were Andrew's camera bag and money-belt and his tripod case, under a humming cloud of flies. The doctor flicked away the end of his cigarette. From a hook behind the door he produced another apron and handed me some surgical gloves. Together we opened the various compartments of the bags, the sergeant noting down our finds. Andrew's camera was there, with a tape inside it. Tapes previously exposed were neatly labelled in their plastic boxes. Batteries, lenses and microphones were all in place, sealed away by the bag's waterproof fabric. The money-belt contained papers and a sodden wedge of francs. Nothing appeared to be missing.

The doctor suggested that we carry out an external examination of the body, and explore the internal organs only if there was evidence of a penetrating wound. We took a deep breath and stepped inside the mortuary. There was no electricity, the only light coming from mesh-covered windows set high along the walls. Andrew's body lay on an autopsy table, under a drip of tepid water from an overhead fitting like a shower nozzle. It did little to dilute the smell, which now had a treacly component from the rum. Andrew's arms had been lowered from the tensed position in which we'd found him, for rigor mortis had long since faded from the muscles. My friend's face was dark and marbled with blood collected in the downward-lying tissues, and the features had slipped from their pressure on the ground; only his thick eyebrows were recognisable. The police doctor and I inspected the clothing all down the front of the body for rips and holes. A right-angled tear in one trouser-leg appeared to have been caused by a thorn. Flies settled on our faces. In the confined space the smell was overpowering. The doctor was evidently suffering too, for he beckoned me outside and we stood in the sunlight, taking great draughts of air until our nausea settled. Then we returned to our work.

Unbuttoned, the shirt-front came away with a sucking sound. I locked my thighs to prevent myself fainting and we continued our inspection over the abdomen and thighs. Holes in the skin we explored with gloved fingers and sounded with probes to measure their depth. No wounds appeared to penetrate the deep fascia, the dense fibrous membrane that sheaths the muscles, nor did the skin-breaks underlie significant tears in the clothing that had covered them. With an assistant's help we turned the body over and continued our inspection. The split in the back of the neck that the commandant had questioned proved superficial, with the strong ligaments that support the head palpably intact; a machete blow would have cut into these structures. It seemed likely that this wound, like the others around the body, were the result of post-mortem depredations by insects or scavengers.

Back at the commandant's office we explained the substance of our findings. There was no sign that Andrew had been the victim of violence, and the police doctor concluded that death might be due to 'natural causes'. Commandant Jean seemed relieved; the hunter could be paid and released. He said that an autopsy report would be drawn up, which I was requested to co-sign as a witness to the accuracy of its contents, and suggested that I return to the headquarters that afternoon to deal with the paperwork and sign that I'd received Andrew's possessions. At the same time he wished to view with me the tape found in Andrew's camera, to see what it might tell us about his last hours.

The film showed images of ordinary beauty, seen though a naturalist's eye. It recorded tiny tree-orchids, two copulating insects that looked like frilly underwear, and a pink aphid and a green aphid trying to pass each other on a slender twig. There were long takes of the edge of the lagoon and wavelets rapping on sand veined with black deposits of titanium dioxide. Andrew had filmed the sunset over the water, indicating that he'd lingered too long on that last visit to the forest and had set out on his return journey to Desirée's vehicle in the dark, when he'd presumably become lost. Every image was imbued with the unbearable poignancy of that knowledge, that these were among the last things that Andrew had seen.

The next afternoon the plane would take Chris, myself and Andrew's body to the capital. In the morning we heard it passing overhead prior to landing, and we went round to make our farewells to Desirée, Mark and the commandant and thank them for their kindness.

'It is good that we could discover your friend and bring him back,' said Commandant Jean, shaking my hand. 'Perhaps we will meet again, and have a drink together, all of us.'

I was back in my room packing when there came a knock at the door. The man outside introduced himself as a journalist on an English national paper. He had flown from London to reach Fort Dauphin on that morning's plane, he explained, in order to interview Chris and I about the search for Andrew, which was the 'lead story' in the UK media. We talked in the car on our way to the airport, Chris answering his questions quietly, though I knew each word must be agonising. The journalist accompanied me round to the aircraft's cargo doors where we watched the fresh-planed casket being loaded. Taking off, we gained height westwards. Chris stared down from her window seat at the green of Petriky Forest as it turned under our wing, and she continued to sit in that wrynecked position of straining to see something long out of sight as the aircraft set its course for Antananarivo.

The ambassador was there to meet us, with the news that a British TV crew was waiting in the arrivals area for an interview. I asked Chris if she'd prefer us to avoid them, but she suggested instead that I use the opportunity to thank all those in England who'd helped with the support and funding of our journey to find Andrew. The film crew behind us, we left the airport and stopped at the roadside before a vista of hills. Chris and the ambassador remained in the car while the cameraman set up. I explained to the TV journalist what Chris had asked me to say, and begged him to avoid the ultimate dickhead interviewer's question: 'How did it feel to find your friend dead?'

It took about three minutes for the man's resolve to be proved useless against the pressures of the medium.

'So, how did it feel,' he blurted, as the cameraman began a slow zoom-in to my features, 'to find your friend dead in the forest?'

In the capital there was much to be arranged. I had long conversations with the assistance company providing Andrew's travel insurance and then with the international undertaker service, entangled in Malagasy bureaucracy while trying to organise the repatriation of his body. The police document I'd co-signed in Fort Dauphin had to be parlayed into a proper death certificate before the deceased could travel, and the state bank required that Andrew's currency declaration form be submitted before his departure and refused to accept that the document had become unreadable and been destroyed. And I fielded requests from London for Andrew's film material, including one coming reportedly from a senior level of the environmental organisation for which Andrew had worked until his departure for Madagascar.

'Everyone's going to run the RTZ story,' was the message relayed to me. 'We must be in front.'

With Andrew's repatriation confirmed for four days hence, Chris proposed that she should wait in Antananarivo to accompany him home while I returned to London on the next available flight. I carried Andrew's tapes in my shoulder bag, entrusted to me, as co-developer of the Madagascar film project, by Chris. Landing in London, I conducted this precious cargo to my flat. A pile of newspaper cuttings relating to the search was on the landing, left by my upstairs neighbour. The light on the answering machine winked like a strobe. I started with my saddest task: calling Andrew's father to tell him what I knew of his son's end. His voice trembled as he thanked me, and again I was seized by a grief that tore my heart. Some hours passed before I felt able to face the telephone messages. Every TV commissioning editor I'd ever worked for wanted to hear from me at once. The most insistent were those who'd never bothered to return my calls when I'd tried to raise interest in our RTZ project months before. Now they wished to discuss a film, budget no problem, about Andrew and Madagascar.

Armed with instructions from Andrew's brothers that his video material was not to be released to anyone until the nature of its usage had been agreed between Chris, the family and myself, I set about calling the various TV editors to let them know I'd received their messages. After years as a scrabbling freelancer it was odd to be in demand. Personal assistants interrupted their bosses' meetings to tell them I was on the line and at once I'd have the editor's hearty tones ringing down the wire, suggesting lunch. I thought of the relish with which Andrew would have greeted this attention to our project. There was a sour pleasure in telling them, with appropriate respect, that they would have to wait in line.

Chris returned and over the following weeks she and I and Andrew's family dealt with the pain of a memorial service and an inquest. At the service many people spoke of Andrew as the fearless, funny, dedicated man I'd known, and enumerated his idiosyncrasies and achievements. Giving evidence at the inquest, I listened to the entomologist eulogise the wonderful relationship that had existed between himself and Andrew in Madagascar, and the environmental organisation director lauding Andrew's selfless commitment. Then the Home Office pathologist took the stand. His findings at a full autopsy, conducted back in England, suggested that death had occurred on the day of Andrew's disappearance or soon thereafter. A full-body X-ray revealed no metal particles from a bullet or a rough blade. No fractures were present, nor evidence of penetrating wounds. Examination of the heart did not reveal signs of coronary artery disease sufficient to suspect a heart attack. The pathologist postulated a biochemical imbalance of body salts from gastroenteritis, along with 'a thermoregulatory derangement of the hyphothalamus', otherwise known as heatstroke. Without a clear cause of death, an 'open verdict' was recorded.

The funeral was held a few days later, in a small country church on a Norfolk hilltop near where Andrew was born. His father was there, an ex-soldier, upright and dignified, and the rest of Andrew's family, along with Chris and her mother and sister. Mist condensed on the leaves of the churchyard yews and shrouded the wetlands around. We stood under a low, cold sky and saw the casket lowered into the ground, and afterwards drank whisky and told stories about Andrew at the wake. Yet he continued to haunt me; not in my dreams, where he walked before me in the forest's green twilight, but rather in the sheer difficulty of trying to get a film made that would be worthy of him.

The meetings that Chris and I attended with commissioning editors were often frustrating. They seemed convinced that there was some thriller element regarding a mining company assassin or a unique moment-of-death video.

'The tape that was in the camera when you found him – what exactly does it show?' they'd ask with prurient fascination. The 'factual entertainment' programmers proposed having a celebrity front the film – a rock personage, a trendy wildlife-show presenter and a green-minded royal were suggested – so that viewers would not be 'put off by the issues'. Now and then Chris and I would hear rumours that negotiations were under way between producers and the environmental organisation director or the entomologist, or receive calls from film-makers who appeared to have an impression that they'd been granted the use of Andrew's tapes for their own Madagascar project. There were long periods when it seemed the documentary would never be made. Eventually, though, a small independent production company managed to interest one of the TV networks in the project and I returned to Fort Dauphin with a minimal crew – a cameraman and a local sound assistant – to start filming.

The *gérant* welcomed me back to my old hotel room overlooking the hulks in the harbour, and enquired sympathetically after Chris. At night on the balcony I watched again the footage Andrew had made on his fateful mission, searching for the essence of my friend through his images. He had left little: a shadow on the grass at the edge of a shot; a voice on the soundtrack; a ghost behind the camera. I set about retracing the journeys he had made along the miles of coast, meeting villagers he'd spoken to and boating through the limpid beauty of the mangroves and lagoons threatened by the dredgers. Petriky remained as it had looked a year before, impenetrable and silent. The villagers still lived in poverty, venturing into the forest for medicinal plants or to hunt or make charcoal, but their paddy fields and fishing grounds and the graves of their ancestors remained thus far untouched. Andrew, dead, was alive for these people. The place where we'd found him was now a shrine, marked out by a pole stockade that kept the forest at bay. A tall rock had been stood there, and a post on which a zebu skull was impaled; sacrificed to Andrew's spirit, which was considered now to be resident in the forest for eternity. The environmental school that Mark ran in Fort Dauphin had a study centre supported by a memorial trust set up in Andrew's name.

The film went out on UK television and we received a call from a Member of Parliament, asking for copies of our research material so that he could ask questions in the House about the ethics of RTZ's operations. Andrew couldn't have hoped for a better outcome. An environmental documentary of the sort we'd first envisaged might have stirred some protest. But his disappearance had shone a spotlight on this remote place, while his death generated discussion of the wider issues – important enough for Andrew to have risked his life here – regarding the right of a global corporation to target a poor country, conduct a high-tech extraction operation employing few locals, repatriate its profits and depart after fifteen years leaving a hole in the ground. The adverse publicity that the mining proposal was attracting, and its marginal benefits for Madagascar, had perhaps made the World Bank reconsider. A decade since Andrew started investigating the RTZ project it remains uninitiated.

But the completion of the documentary left me with an immense emptiness. It was hard to be reconciled to the loss of friends – including Commandant Jean, shot dead in an altercation a month before I'd returned to Fort Dauphin – but most had died far away, and I'd heard only later. I had been so close to accompanying Andrew to Madagascar that I felt I'd been within reach of him in the forest on that last walk. Chopping a path through Petriky in the course of filming, I found myself possessed by a violent urgency, as though, if I were fast enough, I could somehow prevent the thing that had happened a year before. I met the American Peace Corps volunteer working in a small village, humble as any peasant, tending his nursery of shoots that would restore the eroded hill-forest. He confirmed the account of Andrew handing over his medical kit and still felt guilty, wondering whether the tablets and rehydration solution could have saved Andrew's life. I knew, though, that the fault was mine. I was the one experienced in bush medicine, in tropical illness, in emergency resuscitation. And instead of saving my friend I had left him alone in that most absolute wilderness, of solitary death. I did not know how to find expiation.

8

Bullet Rash

My first patient was eight months' pregnant. She was anaemic from malnutrition and she had a fever, probably from malaria. But then almost everyone in Kuito was malnourished – the people of this small town in Angola's central highlands had been on siege rations for two years – and malaria was endemic. The reason she was lying on a stretcher in the shell-damaged emergency room of Kuito's hospital was that she'd been caught in a UNITA attack in the small hours of the morning. A bullet had entered through the back of her neck, passing forward and out through the left side of her face. A rough dressing covered the exit wound. From beneath it seeped a sheen of pink. The woman was mute, from pain or shock, and responded to our voices with a stunned slowness that made it difficult to assess her awareness. The visible part of her face was frozen in an expression of unremitting horror.

Kuito was in its twenty-sixth year of war. Since 1975, when the Angolan conflict started, the town had been contested: overrun by the rebels of UNITA, recaptured by the army and fought over street by street. Recently the rebels had been pushed back by government forces so that the official front extended in a curve about thirty miles to the south-east. Road links to the garrisons at Andulo in the north and Huambo to the west were under tenuous daytime control by the Angolan army, but a UNITA counteroffensive was under way and at night ambushes and attacks occurred well inside the front line. Kuito's security perimeter extended only to the edges of the *barrios* – the shanty settlements thrown up by war-displaced villagers – a few miles in each direction from the main street. Beyond, the bullets flew.

There were two others caught in the attack that wounded the pregnant woman. One I never saw; she was left dead at the scene.

The other was a man who'd received a burst from an AK-47 assault rifle through his legs, shattering the bone. It had taken hours to bring the victims over rough roads to Kuito hospital, and when they were unloaded it was evident that he had bled to death in the back of the truck. We took the survivor straight to surgery. Beneath her dressing the damage was horrific. All that remained of the eye was a pit of shredded tissue. The anaesthetic nurse was anxious about using Ketamine on a pregnant woman – it can cause uterine contractions and premature labour – but we had no other means of putting our patient to sleep, so she injected the drug into the drip-line. At once the woman suffered a respiratory arrest, a crisis for her unborn baby. The anaesthetist pressed a mask onto her face and pumped in oxygen, but it bubbled out through the ruined eye: the bullet had blown out the bone that separates the nasal space from the inner side of the eye socket. The pulse-oximeter alarm chimed as the oxygen level in her blood began to drop. I packed wet gauze into the hole in her face, trying to block the route through which the life-saving oxygen was escaping. Eventually she coughed and gagged and started breathing again and we could continue the operation.

Acute war surgery is crude but straightforward: stop the bleeding, cut away dead and lacerated tissue. I stretched the ruptured eyeball over my finger-tip and snipped away the muscular attachments until it remained connected only by the optic nerve, which I tied and divided. Then I picked out fragments of bone from the shattered wall of the eye socket and tried to reconstruct it with muscle and flesh. The woman's face was hugely swollen from blood that had tracked into the tissues and her nostrils leaked clear cerebro-spinal fluid, indicating that the bullet had torn the membranes protecting the brain. Meningitis seemed inevitable; it was difficult to know whether she would live. I dressed the wound while the Angolan *técnico médico* wrote up the operation notes in Portuguese and prescribed intravenous antibiotics. From overhead came the roar of circling transport planes, the clatter of a military helicopter.

✛

The Kuito enclave was cut off from the rest of the country except by air. Without the eight daily supply flights by the United

Nations World Food Programme, the place could not have held out. UNITA knew this, and – equipped with ground-to-air missiles – periodically targeted aid aircraft. Two United Nations transports had been blown out of the skies near Kuito within days of each other, around the start of 1999. The story I'd heard included an additional tragedy. The second plane carried a son trying to find out what had happened to his father, who had been on the first aircraft to go missing; his flight disappeared in the same way, with no survivors. This precarious air-bridge remained the only way to get into Kuito from the Angolan capital.

I was here with my photographer friend Guy, who'd been recording the Angolan conflict for years. He had hopped many aid flights in and out of its war-torn towns, and at Luanda Airport I had tried to emulate his relaxed stroll as we walked along the line of green-and-yellow-camouflaged ground attack aircraft of the Força Aérea do Angola, rocket pods under their wings, being refuelled on the concrete apron.

Our transport plane had flown a lot of miles. The white paint was sun blistered and smudged with oil, the 'UN' on its fuselage faded to grey. As we took off in a vibrating blur, roaring over the patchwork slums around the runway's end, I remembered the words of the South African Airways captain when my flight from Johannesburg had arrived here a few days before.

'We have just landed at Luanda International Airport,' he'd announced. 'For your own safety we recommend that you remain seated until the aircraft has come to a complete stop and then stay aboard and take the return flight to South Africa. Thank you.'

For the UN pilots this sortie was routine, requiring only standard ground-fire avoidance procedures. We followed the rise of the shadowed highlands from the coastal plain, climbing and climbing. At maximum altitude, with Kuito visible as a smudge on the dark plateau, the aircraft stood on one wingtip and began a corkscrew dive that pressed us into our seats. Far below, the airfield's oily streak – its runway haloed by zigzag trench lines – whirled like a spinning clock-hand around a grid of streets that enlarged with each rotation. Columns of smoke slanted above the land to the east where the front line lay.

Our descent was precisely calculated, so that a twitch of the controls flipped us out of our spiral in perfect alignment to land. The wheels slammed over the cratered runway and we bounced past dugouts and artillery pieces and the burned-out shell of an attack helicopter. At the end of the runway a wrecked Antonov transport plane was reared up on its tail so that wings and fuselage formed a great metal cross; a symbol of grand ruin. In its shadow waited a group of white vehicles belonging to aid organisations based in the town, who'd come to meet the flight. Many of them knew Guy, who was greeted warmly; not many visitors came to Kuito out of choice. We threw our bags into the back of a pick-up, climbed up after them and the convoy set off along the strip of ragged black-top that led through the refugee shacks back to town.

Army trucks travelled the other way, packed with troops who swayed in unison over the ruts and potholes. Children scattered at the blast of their horns into the mango trees beside the road and one-legged men, empty trouser legs flapping, swung themselves up onto the verge on agile crutches. At the entrance to the town a concrete welcome-arch leaned askew. The buildings that flanked the main avenue were eroded by shellfire, entire rooms excavated from their facades. Trees along the boulevard had been sheared off a yard from the ground. A block of apartments was folded at one end so that its floors converged like a collapsed accordion, but people appeared to be living in the tilted ruin and the irregular gaps in the wall were draped with sacking. Villas were roofless, their walls pocked with a confluent rash of bullet holes. Grave-mounds and crosses stood in the overgrown gardens.

This had once been a prosperous town. Founded around 1870 as administrative capital of the province of Bíe, Kuito boomed in the 1950s when Portugal's dictator Salazar declared his imperial vision of *Estado Novo,* the New State, whose colonies would be 'overseas provinces' of the motherland. Tens of thousands of farm-ers were shipped out from Portugal's overworked soil in order to establish a settler economy – fruit and coffee plantations – in the fertile Angolan highlands. The Ministry of Agricultural Planning for the entire colonial empire was centralised at Nova Lisboa, capi-tal of the neighbouring province of Huambo, and both towns lay on the route of the Benguela railway that was to open up the African interior by connecting the Atlantic coast to the Indian Ocean.

Most of Kuito had been built in the following twenty years, of pre-stressed concrete that lent itself to soaring cantilevers and Deco curves. The material had proved remarkably resilient to gunfire. Bullets and shell fragments perforated it through and through and the walls showed the path of every splinter from the radiating bursts of rocket-propelled grenades. Even direct hits with high explosive were absorbed by the elasticity of the internal reinforcing iron, leaving structures warped but standing, their fractured concrete laced together on metal stalks. A dry water-feature lined in turquoise tiles cascaded down the axis of the square. Two bronze nymphs, one bare-breasted, the other coyly lowering her bikini bottom, graced plinths within the empty pool. Though the tiles were gouged by shrapnel the bronze girls remained exquisitely intact.

'There is no crisis in Kuito,' announced Colin, the district head of an Irish humanitarian organisation based in the town. 'Just the same old emergency that's been under way for years and is currently going through one of its regular flare-ups.'

He spread out a map and weighted its corners with deactivated anti-personnel mines, their plastic cases designed to be difficult to find by mine detectors. The Angolan army's advance to the southeast, Colin explained, had captured settlements which they now held – with fierce artillery exchanges – as part of the Kuito enclave's perimeter. Villagers fleeing the fighting were flooding into the government-held sector.

'One could be forgiven for becoming a mite cynical about our work.' Colin scratched his beard. 'The offensive is intended to deny food to the rebels by dispersing the people who feed them. The Angolan government can do this knowing that the aid organisations will take responsibility for the displaced, so when we step in and help them we're in effect supporting the army's strategy.'

At the same time, he continued, UNITA appeared to be pillaging all the food they could from the populace; grave malnutrition was evident among those reaching government lines. These highland people were Ovimbundu, the tribe from which UNITA leader Jonas Savimbi drew his support. Their suffering had started in the

'First War' following the 1975 Portuguese pull-out, when South Africa invaded Angola to stop the Marxist MPLA forming the country's new government, and was turned back by an airlift of Cuban soldiers. Angola became a Cold War battleground, with the MPLA receiving Soviet arms and Cuban advisors while South Africa and the US transformed Savimbi's guerrilla band into an armed presence across central Angola. Attacks for which UNITA claimed credit were generally the work of South African forces operating from neighbouring South West Africa, but President Reagan was sufficiently impressed by Savimbi's anti-communist stance to describe UNITA as 'the moral equivalent of the Founding Fathers'. Sophisticated Stinger ground-to-air missiles were supplied to his forces through Zaïre, via the assistance of America's other great friend in the region, the monstrously corrupt President Mobutu. Angolan government control became restricted to the major towns, with road-travel disrupted by ambushes and military and aid flights knocked from the skies. Angolan independence seemed stillborn.

UNITA lost its southern supporter in 1990 when South Africa withdrew from South West Africa, which became independent Namibia. The next year, pressure from the US and post-Soviet Russia forced UNITA and the MPLA to agree to a UN-supervised demobilisation programme and elections. International agencies flooded into the ravaged country to restore basic services: health, education, water supplies. Transport links were reopened to regions that had long been cut off from aid. But Savimbi denounced the 1992 election results as fraudulent – he'd believed his foreign advisors who had promised a UNITA victory – and took the country back to war. The people of Kuito had voted eighty percent for UNITA, but this did not spare them. Reconstruction was abandoned and aid staff evacuated as Kuito's 'Second War' began, a nine-month siege from January to September 1993. The rebels captured one side of the main avenue which became the front line, with government forces holding an area of ten blocks in the eastern part of the city. UNITA shelled the enclave relentlessly, a thousand projectiles landing daily through the worst months of the siege. People ate grass and banana roots. Parties of desperate civilians stole through UNITA lines to find food, losing one in three to land mines and gunfire. Around thirty thousand townspeople died from wounds, disease and hunger and were buried at night – to avoid UNITA snipers – in yards and gardens, interred under piles of rubble.

In 1994 UNITA was forced back by an Angolan army offensive and aid agencies returned to Kuito with emergency assistance that gradually gave way to development and rehabilitation projects. But new UN-sponsored peace talks in 1998, aimed at creating an MPLA/UNITA coalition government, also failed, and by mid-December the "Third War" was under way. UNITA forces approached to within a few miles of the town and pounded it for three months with rockets and artillery, and when the aid organisations returned in 1999 it was to find their projects in ruins. Airlifting in medicine, food and shelter materials, they'd spent the last two years rebuilding what had been destroyed.

The situation now, explained Colin, was what the Kuito aid workers called 'stable instability'. Civilians displaced by the fighting were entering the government-held enclave in large numbers, ill and starving, with humanitarian agencies trucking the most malnourished of these IDPs – internally displaced persons – to therapeutic feeding centres in the town. Their convoys had been curtailed, however, following an ambush the day before.

'You'd better see the latest security briefing,' he said, extracting a document from a file.

'There is evidence of substantial enemy movement across the province from south to north, rendering travel on the roads around Kuito open to risk,' it began. In the past three days there had been an attack on a convoy to the west of town on the Huambo road, with three trucks burned and seven dead. Ten miles from Kuito an army engineer had been killed by a new-laid mine while returning along a strip of road he'd just cleared. A rebel attack on Camacupa burned four houses, while a tripwire device had caused carnage near Chipeta twelve miles to the east. Attacks on villages along the roads to Andulo and Chitembo were bringing many civilian casualties.

'It's not always clear who's doing the shooting,' Colin said. 'If you ask the people who attacked them they'll say *os enemigos:* the enemy. It's wisest not to say anything against the security forces.'

The wounded, the sick and the critically malnourished ended up at Kuito's hospital, the only one functioning in the government-controlled enclave. It was run by a handful of personnel from Médecines sans Frontières (Doctors Without Borders), the international relief organisation whose operations have provided the model for successful humanitarian medical intervention around the world. In the thirteen years that the group had operated in Kuito its staff had needed evacuation nine times: sometimes for a week or two, but for months on end during the sieges. MSF had offices in a patched-up house near the hospital, to which I made my way through the glaring afternoon light. Banners hung from the ruins: the Angolan Movement of Women (silhouette of a woman with a shouldered rifle), the Organisation of Ex-Combatants. In the MSF office I introduced myself to Danny, the group's medical co-ordinator, explaining that I was here by default; an arranged mission – in which Guy and I would have flown into the airfield of Andulo to the north with a load of humanitarian aid – had fallen through, and we'd been delivered instead to Kuito via the UN food flight. Arriving thus unexpectedly, I wondered whether there might be some medical work I could help with at the hospital.

'You are welcome.' Danny shook my hand doubtfully. 'The hospital, yes... well, it may not be like hospitals you are used to. It was smashed in 1993 and then smashed all over again two years ago. We are trying to get things going again. It's very basic: over-crowded, few drugs, lots of disease and malnutrition, plus the wounded.'

'I've actually worked with your organisation before,' I said. 'During the war in Mozambique.' I explained how I'd arrived in a small coastal town and been pressed into service at their hospital to fill in for the surgeon who was away.

'You're a surgeon?' Danny beamed, pumping my hand. 'You are really very welcome; in fact, you have no idea how fortuitous your arrival. Our surgeon has been on duty day and night-time for ten weeks and she needs a break. We were deciding to fly her back to the capital for some days to relax.' Danny hesitated. 'Is it possible that you could...'

'Of course,' I said, swallowing hard. 'No problem.'

Despite previous assignments in Kurdistan, Burma and Mozambique, I was hardly prepared for taking over as the sole surgeon of a war zone hospital. The year before, I had been in Eritrea when a massive offensive by neighbouring Ethiopia broke the Eritrean front line. I'd offered my assistance in hospitals overwhelmed by mass casualties coming straight from the fighting. The war had been under way for two years – and, apart from a five-year break, for thirty years before that – and the Eritrean surgeons were very experienced. Under their guidance I was able to do the work demanded of me, though I'd wondered whether each case might be more than I could cope with. Now I would be on my own, dealing with wounds to chest and limbs and belly for which I feared that my skills and knowledge would not be adequate. No matter how many times I have lifted the knife and taken that step into uncertainty, I've never become used to it. But the possession of surgical training is a responsibility that cannot be sidestepped. Following Danny's directions I set off down the road, skirting a compound of armoured vehicles with UN markings, some carrying the marks of bullet strikes on their white-painted sides. At the hospital entrance an ambulance ground past me through the sand to stop at the much pock-marked *banco de urgencia*, the emergency room, from which some nurses emerged to help the crew struggle up the steps with their loaded stretcher.

The hospital's front had recently been patched and a smart red cross painted on a corner of the façade, but the rest of its walls were cross-hatched with fragmentation scars, grey against the pink plaster. The surgical wards opened off a long veranda. Inside, rounds were in progress. A slow waft of air through the glassless windows circulated flies and the reek of sepsis. Children and adults lay on bare beds or on rubber mattresses or reed mats on the floor, their afflictions – burns, incisions, purulent abscesses – unbandaged for inspection. In the midst of this carnival stood a young woman, the only foreigner present. She looked to be in her early thirties, slender and clear-featured. I realised she was the surgeon I would temporarily be replacing.

'I'm Rosa,' she said, shaking my hand. 'Danny just called me on the radio. Thanks for your offer to help.' She introduced me to Jesùs and Eduardo; Angolan *técnicos médicos* – medical technicians – trained in basic surgery. The *technicos* explained that they had been concerned about major trauma cases arriving while Doctora Rosa was absent; now, they said graciously, their worries were at an end. I thanked them in my clumsy Portuguese, hoping that their confidence was justified.

The range of pathology around us did little to reassure me. Abdominal cases included gunshot wounds, intestinal perforations from typhoid and bladder damage following obstetric complications. Beds were occupied by women who'd required Caesarean sections for problem deliveries. A six-year-old girl sobbed endlessly; an infected fracture of her leg would not heal and the bone had been laid open from knee to ankle to help it drain, the long wound cupping a froth of pus. Yes, confirmed Rosa, these were all our patients, for there was only one surgeon to do all the operating in this place, and that included obstetrics and orthopaedic surgery.

'Head injuries also come to us,' she said, indicating an old woman just brought in, found unconscious in the street. I examined the frail figure who hardly indented the rubber mattress. A great, doughy collection of blood under the scalp suggested the likelihood of a fractured skull. I tried to check her pupils for the dilation that could indicate brain damage, but the cheeks and eyelids were so swollen from bruising that her eyes could not be seen.

'We can only wait and see if she wakes up,' said Rosa. 'We have no X-ray to take pictures of the skull and no facilities for neurosurgery.'

'Who could have beaten her like this?' I asked.

Rosa shrugged. 'Anyone. There is so much violence here, because of the war.' She looked around the circle of wounds and maimed, limbs and stumps upraised like a convention of beggars. 'There is never enough suffering.'

Until Rosa left the next afternoon, we worked together at the hospital. A full list of patients awaited surgery. I joined Eduardo in the operating theatre. The man on the table had lost his right hand and great bites of his thighs to the explosion of a grenade. His wrist ended in cusps of cartilage, splayed like petals, all that remained of the hand after flesh and bones had been blown away. We tried a forearm amputation but through our incision the muscles bulged black and dead, crumbling between the jaws of the clamps. We cut higher and higher, trying to find the place where the skin edges bled briskly, indicating an adequate circulation for healing. Eventually we were forced to take the arm off above the elbow. Muscles were divided, vessels tied, and the saw-wire sang through the ivory bone.

In the adjacent operating room Rosa had received the next case, a woman who'd been in labour for forty-eight hours before being brought to hospital. She had no measurable blood pressure; we struggled to locate a vein to start an intravenous infusion and eventually used one in her neck. The uterus felt misshapen and we couldn't hear the baby's heartbeat, and – most worryingly – the catheter I passed into her bladder drained not urine but blood. We scrubbed our hands with gritty soap and gloved up. The diagnosis was confirmed at surgery: the uterus was ruptured and the child, when we brought it out, had not survived. The tear through the front of the womb had gone into her bladder. As we repaired the laceration, blood continued to well up from torn uterine vessels that proved impossible to oversew. Eventually it was necessary to remove the whole womb – a hysterectomy – in order to stop the bleeding and save the woman's life.

Then it was time for Rosa to go. I walked her out to the truck waiting to take her to the airfield, but on our way through the *banco de urgencia* we checked a patient waiting for surgical assessment. She'd come from the IDP camp, a woman in her sixties with abdominal pain and her spleen enlarged to four or five times its normal size – probably the result of chronic malaria – so that it filled the left side of her abdomen like a firm loaf. The pain could be a sign that the spleen was about to rupture, a surgical emergency, so we put up a drip-line and admitted her for observation. Then Rosa was gone and I was the only surgeon in Kuito, responsible – with the able *technicos* – for the resident population of a hundred and sixty thousand civilians plus a similar number of displaced persons in camps around the town, and whatever military casualties found their way to our door.

✚

The woman with the blown-out eye had been my first patient. The next was a man from another part of the battlefield who'd been shot through the top of his thigh close to the major vessels, and I had to explore his wound to see whether these were intact. The bullet had also torn through his scrotum, leaving one testicle exposed like a dull pearl. Its blood supply seemed intact so I restored it to its ragged pouch, closing the skin around a rubber tube that would be removed once any pus had drained. Then I operated on a young woman with an infected abdominal surgery wound that had burst open beneath the blankets while she was lying on the ward, exposing bowel and putting her into septic shock. Her condition was too unstable to tolerate being put to sleep, so I injected skin and muscle with local anaesthetic and re-stitched her belly. Further cases accumulated steadily: abscesses to be opened and drained, fractures needing setting, a man with his shoulder-blade shattered by a rifle-shot.

Every day brought a fresh tide of casualties. Jesùs and Eduardo would start the morning by writing the day's operating list on a board in the operating department, but every hour or two it needed revision as new patients arrived, the severity of their problems dictating the priority for surgery. Between operations we would go to the wards to examine patients on whom a surgical opinion had been requested. One night Eduardo and I visited the maternity unit to assess a woman admitted with abdominal pain. The corridors were in darkness – the hospital generator's power was limited – and inside the ward a neon tube shed a dim green light. On the delivery table a woman was in labour, a midwife beside her. Beyond lay our patient, on a mattress on the floor. Her skin radiated heat that could be felt from inches away, despite the day's warmth still hanging in the ward. Fever and flank tenderness suggested a kidney infection – rather than a tubal pregnancy – as the likely diagnosis, and we prescribed antibiotics and medication for her pain. While we were examining her the woman on the delivery table began to give birth. She made no sound, only turning her eyes up to the ceiling with the intensity of her contractions. The head appeared and then the baby was out with a splash and a slither, being wrapped by the midwife in a towel. Its mother stood up, naked but for a cloth that she held between her thighs. In the low light her body gleamed with sweat as she walked past us to her bed, as steady and sure-footed as though on her way to collect water.

✛

Beyond the hospital stood rows of canvas barrack-tents, the critical feeding centre for the most severely malnourished IDPs. This was a grim place, where flies clustered around the eyes of faces pared back to the shape of the underlying bone. Most were children, some alone – separated from their parents in the panic of the attack that had driven them from their villages – others cradled by exhausted mothers. They had been hiding in the bush for days before they reached help, and were in a desperate state. Intensive treatment with intravenous fluid and milk and protein supplement, plus drugs for respiratory infections and dysentery, did not prevent around a quarter of them dying. Some of the survivors haunted the hospital corridors or congregated at night in the shadows near the outdoor kitchen where cauldrons of maize porridge bubbled on wood fires. The kids all looked the same: stick limbs, dusty hair, their eyes downcast. They avoided physical contact and did not respond to conversation, moving on the edge of vision like sidling shades. After a while one stopped noticing them. It was difficult to imagine their future.

Angola had many ghosts: of the million-plus people that the war had killed, of the hundred and seventy-six thousand children under the age of five who'd died in the previous year alone of disease and malnutrition. There were also the phantasms created by humanitarian aid. Around a third of Angola's twelve million population were war-displaced, and the UN food flights into Kuito fed some two hundred thousand of them. It was useless simply to toss food into a forest of outstretched hands: the needy had to be located, collected in some sort of settlement and registered so that rations could be systematically distributed. This was a huge task in which many aid groups collaborated, supplying shelter materials, water, food, vaccination programmes and even – from those agencies with a long-term view – development projects to encourage the return of self-sufficiency. Sometimes on the edges of the *barrios* around Kuito new suburbs of mud and straw would spring up overnight, built by IDPs already registered elsewhere, in an attempt to obtain a second monthly ration that might ensure family survival, while allowing the surplus to be turned to profit. The job of catching these phantom refugees – in midnight house-to-house raids to check identities – fell upon the same humanitarian workers whose task it was to feed the displaced.

The war seemed eternal, its resolution lost in a mist of blood and famine. Even after the demise of Savimbi's main supply route, when Mobutu fell from power in Zaïre in 1997, UNITA had continued to find arms and equipment. When the Angolan government provided military backing for the Democratic Republic of Congo's new president, Laurent Kabila, UNITA had made common cause with the rebel forces marshalled against Kabila, opening a new front south of the Congolese capital Kinshasa. With South African–arranged peace talks under way between the factions, the UNITA forces – freshly re-equipped – were returning to Angola. They had also bought new weapons on the open market, funded by the more than one hundred million dollars the rebel group obtained yearly from its control of Angola's northern diamond fields. An international treaty to control the flow of 'conflict diamonds' had foundered on the failure of some diamond-trading countries – Zambia, the Central African Republic and Israel – to co-operate. Meantime UNITA had begun a major offensive across Angola, with attacks close to Luanda. In response Angolan government forces were being rapidly re-armed, the revenue coming from the oil wells of Cabinda Province where the international corporations Gulf, Chevron and Elf pumped out a hundred thousand barrels a day.

Despite the precariousness of the situation – there had been two recent explosions in Kuito blamed on UNITA bombs, and the growing battle to the south-east had the aid organisations drawing up contingency plans to close down their projects and pull out their personnel within forty-eight hours – there was among the residents of Kuito and its *barrios* an enormous pressure for normality. People gathered for services in roofless churches, children attended class in the open beside destroyed schools. Opposite the ruined cinema the Esplanade Bar was back in business, plastic sheeting draping its rafters. Shrubs in the main square had been clipped into neat spheres. Even the town's central marketplace was thriving. The coffee trees planted by the Portuguese were still producing and hand-ground beans were on sale, the crop so rich that it could be smelled right across the other side of the warren of stalls. The peasant farmers with their little pyramids of tomatoes were jostled by sellers of American cigarettes and Johnny Walker, brought in as supercargo on the military flights to Andulo.

A number of the entrepreneurs were *mutiladas* – women amputees – who had lost legs to mines. Colin's agency provided them small loans for self-help projects; the women's groups used the money to buy bulk staples (often from food aid supplies), which they re-packaged and sold in smaller amounts at a provisions market on an open space beyond the hospital. Previously a football field, it had become a cemetery during the last siege and the grave mounds now formed the counters of impromptu stalls. For male amputees – mainly ex-soldiers – there were fewer options. The government in whose service they'd been wounded did little to help them; these *mutilados* lived in the derelict, rocket-ruined shell of the Ministry of Education building, drawing rations according to the generosity of the garrison's quartermaster. The most enterprising among them had cornered the shoeshine trade in the central market and sat all day in attendance on those that had both feet, but business was difficult, for only a tiny part of the town's population could afford shoes. In their spare time the amputees brought to a high gloss the pristine shoe that encased their artificial foot: these lasted much longer than the one on the living leg, so that few of them owned a matching pair.

✪

New mine victims arrived constantly at the hospital. One ward was filled with them, civilian and military, in army jackets or the bright-patterned *capulanas* worn by the women. I had never seen a person step on a mine, but once in Ovamboland in northern Namibia I'd heard the explosion and the bellowing of a cow in the scrub, and I had watched from the path as it tried to get up and fell, and tried to get up and fell, while the herdsman went off to borrow a rifle to shoot it. I could sense the animal's bewilderment that suddenly it had lost that instinctive, obvious ability to stand, and I imagined that humans, unless they were killed outright by the explosion, would also keep trying to get up, uncomprehendingly, like animals.

Perhaps the young soldier I was examining could be described as lucky. He'd survived the blast of the anti-personnel mine and the evacuation from the front, been dropped at our *banco de urgencia* rather than the military hospital – which I'd heard was always short of supplies – and now he lay on a bed in the ward with some morphine inside him. When he looked down both his legs were there. But I knew that the right one was as good as gone: the heel blown off, the tibia splintered and the lower part of the calf already taking on that tense, dusky look that indicates a disrupted blood supply. In the Western hospitals where I'd learned my art we would have immobilised the fracture within a steel frame and performed an angiogram X-ray to identify points of vessel damage in order to bypass them with graft operations and restore circulation. But there were no facilities here to perform an angiogram even if we'd had the nursing care available to tend an open fracture on the pus-stinking ward, and so my training as an arterial surgeon was useless to save his leg and we took him to the operating room and cut it off.

Ketamine anaesthesia produces excellent pain-block but suppresses consciousness only partly, so that patients sometimes show a puzzled semi-wakefulness as though aware of what is happening to them. We swathed the foot in a green surgical drape to seal away the shattered heel. As we lifted the leg to wrap a drape around the tourniquet at the top of the thigh, it rose of its own volition, so that the soldier appeared to be offering it to me. He lifted his head a little and I looked away, concentrating on the surgery so I would not know if he was watching my hands as I worked. The first task was to form flaps of skin and muscle; longer than the length of bone, in order that they would come together over its end to form the stump. I made the front incision across the shin, eight inches below the lower edge of the kneecap. Healthy skin parted under the knife, a violation of my instinct to make better. Then, beginning on the inner aspect of the leg, I swept the blade round the back of the calf in a downward curve through skin and fascia and living muscle and up again to meet the end of the front cut on the leg's outer side. Even now it would not be too late to go back to try to undo the damage and save the leg, but there were other casualties waiting and new wounded on their way, and this was no place for complex surgery.

The nerves were divided next, each one drawn down into the wound and cut cleanly so that the severed end retracted up into the flesh. I dissected out arteries and veins, the very structures I had been trained to preserve and restore, and crushed each with a clamp before dividing it, tying my suture tightly around the vessel so that it would not slip off and cause a fatal haemorrhage. Using an osteotome – a blunt-edged chisel – I scraped the periosteal membrane upwards from the bone's surface, pushing the meat and sinew above the place that the cut would be made. Now nothing remained to join the patient to his lower leg but the bare bone. The saw-teeth bit through the slender wand of the fibula with a few strokes. Then the hefty tibia: first an oblique slice into the shin, angled back and down, then, slightly lower, another cut straight across the shaft so that it passed through the first saw-line and removed a triangular chip of bone to bevel the tibia's sharp front edge. The saw was blunt – we did so many amputations – and my wrist became tired. Eduardo took over while I steadied the leg. The last bridge of bone was separated. The amputated limb felt suddenly as heavy as lead in my arms, heavier than an entire body; the stump, freed of its weight, bounded upwards.

The anaesthetist loosened the tourniquet and blood flowed from the cut flesh. We oversewed oozing vessels and poured on sterile water to wash out clot ands debris that might lead to gangrene. Despite this cleansing we knew that dirt remained in the wound, blasted up by the force of the mine's explosion, and in order to permit the discharge of inevitable infection, the flaps of skin and muscle were tacked together with a single loose stitch around a rubber drain. As Eduardo carried away the cut-off limb, wrapped in a drape, its owner's head turned slowly, his gaze appearing to follow it as it was borne past.

If he survived the post-operative sepsis, his stump would be rebandaged daily to help it heal. Then he'd swing down the hill on his crutches to the prosthetic limb factory at the Red Cross *Centro de Ortopedia,* the only industry in Kuito. The engineer who ran the place had shown me around. First a cast of the stump was made in the measuring room. A sheet of brown plastic, heated in a special oven, was vacuum-moulded to its shape and lined with padding. Around this the limb was constructed – with a steel knee-joint if needed, depending on the level of the amputation – and fitted with a black rubber foot. Limb components were stacked on shelves, along with arms and hands of tan-coloured nylon manufactured in Red Cross workshops in Cambodia. I was reminded of the anti-personnel mines in Colin's office, made in Russia and Kuwait and Italy of similar dull shades of plastic. The artificial limb industry, like the manufacture of land mines, was an example of successful globalisation.

Over the course of its long war Angola has been estimated to have suffered a hundred thousand victims of land mines. For each survivor of a mine explosion another died – either quickly through blood-loss or as a result of infection – but that still left Angola with the highest percentage of amputees of any country in the world, and a heritage of buried explosives that would take a hundred years to clear; foot by foot, as the joke went. The end of fighting, when people returned to the lands to grow their first crops of peace, would see a terrible harvest. A miracle would be needed, along the lines of the genetically modified plant I'd heard about that was supposedly being engineered for seeding over conflict zones. Quick-growing, its roots were designed to be sensitive to the presence of tiny parts-per-billion concentrations of chemical molecules from explosive compounds that leached into the soil; these would cause the leaves to grow red instead of green, marking the position of each mine. But its deployment in Angola would be years away, if indeed the plant even existed. In the meantime the rains washed mines onto tracks previously cleared, new ones were being planted by UNITA and by government forces and minefields remained unmapped, causing indiscriminate casualties.

To replenish their ranks, soldiers and police combed the streets and *barrios,* grabbing every man they could. Police trucks drove by, their beds packed with frightened-looking boys in blue caps just inducted into the force. The army press-gangs tied their captives' T-shirts together front and back to form a chain and ran them through the town between files of sweating soldiers. Drivers and translators employed by the aid groups were caught up in these hunts, forcing the heads of the organisations to apply at military headquarters to try to get them released. At night there was gunfire in the town and – somewhere at the edge of hearing – the rumble of the bombardment. Kuito had no electricity. Sounds echoed in the blacked-out streets; it was difficult to assess how far away they were. Aid staff were forbidden to walk anywhere after dark, so when I finished working late I was driven in a hospital truck to the house that Guy and I shared. One night I was awoken by a pounding at the door. Light shone through the holes in the metal panel (relic of a mortar shell that had landed on the front step), projecting a frieze of wavering shapes into the hall. Eduardo, accompanied by an armed guard, had come to take me to the hospital; there was a case of *traumatismo de bala* – bullet wound – in the emergency room.

The patient was ten years old.

'This is Maria,' said Jesùs. 'Her name in the Kimbundu language is *Cafilé;* it means "the one who has survived". Maybe her mother had lost children before her.'

Maria sat forward on the edge of the couch, each breath a grunt of pain. She had been shot though her left side, the bullet exiting about four inches round to her back. I was hoping that it had not damaged abdominal organs – her intestines gurgled normally and her urine contained no blood – but the pain prevented her relaxing her stomach muscles enough for me to make a proper assessment. The only finding, through my stethoscope, was an absence of breath-sounds in the left half of her chest: the lung had collapsed, and we needed to insert a chest drain that would allow it to re-expand. Though alone and frightened – she'd been brought to the hospital before her parents had been located – Maria showed an extra-ordinary composure.

She sat still on the operating table while I injected local anaesthetic around the holes, front and back. They bubbled and sucked a froth of blood with each breath. Quickly I trimmed the skin-edges and stitched the wounds before turning my attention to the drain. Below her armpit I injected anaesthetic between the ribs, through skin and muscle. The needle passed through the pleura – the sensitive membrane lining the chest cavity – with a pop, making her gasp. I cut with a scalpel through the numb area. The new wound whistled air and I plugged it with a finger while I readied the plastic drain tube to pass along the track made by the blade. Maria coughed and cried as it slid into her chest. I stitched the drain to her skin to prevent it being dislodged and then attached it to a tube that ran down into a bottle standing on the floor. Half filled with water, this formed a simple one-way valve; as she exhaled, air bubbled from the submerged end of the tube, allowing the lung, by increments, to re-expand. Maria began breathing more easily, though she still flinched with each inhalation. I wished I could speak to her to allay her fear, but my Portuguese, gleaned from doctoring in Mozambique and Brazil, was mostly medical terminology and quite inadequate to comfort a child. We prescribed antibiotics and painkillers and reassessment in the morning.

Riding back to my sleeping quarters, I stood with the guard in the back of the truck as we travelled through the deserted streets. I offered him a cigarette and lit one myself. Having stopped smoking some years before, I had started again in Kuito, partly because of the shortage of food – the aid flights brought in only sixty-five percent of the populace's calorie needs, and tobacco is an efficient suppressor of hunger – and also because values here were inverted; amidst all the risks attendant on the war, cigarettes seemed positively safe, while tasting specially luxurious with comforts so scarce. Exhaling, I gazed up at the arc of stars and the bright constellation of the Southern Cross, and considered the seduction of working in places like this, that if continued for too long made one unsuited to anything else. I wondered if I might become like those burned-out doctors I had met in the field whom they keep trying to send home but who keep coming back; getting flakier, going native, losing their edge, until one day they are unable to beat the next attack of malaria or don't hit the floor fast enough to avoid an incoming shell.

☧

When I reached the hospital the next morning Rosa was back, earlier than expected. She had found Luanda exhausting, the superficiality of people's pre-occupations in the city intolerable. Together we assessed Maria's condition. Breath-sounds over her left lung indicated that it had re-inflated, but now her belly was distended. We decided that we had to operate. The blade cut easily through her thin abdominal muscles. Inside, some blood lay between the folds of bowel; not an encouraging sign. Searching the belly – our retractors were too small, and the spleen, enlarged from malaria, was in the way – we found a hole in the deepest part of the diaphragm, through which Rosa extracted a chip of rib. The top of the spleen bore a laceration that miraculously had stopped bleeding. Rosa's deft assistance made it possible to for me stitch the ragged edge of diaphragm that billowed with each breath, and after a shared struggle the defect was closed. The lung, which had collapsed again during the operation, began to re-expand.

Afterwards we went around the crowded surgical wards to assess the other patients. The chaos that had overwhelmed me on my arrival at the hospital was replaced by a sense of order. The man whose thigh I'd operated on was doing well, and the woman with the destroyed eye was alive and talking – my improvised repair of the socket appeared to be healing, and her pregnancy seemed healthy – though she was still on intravenous antibiotics to prevent meningitis. The hysterectomy case had been discharged. But not every outcome was happy. A woman awaiting surgery for a bladder injury had died overnight, from causes that were not apparent. The little girl with the infected fracture that wouldn't heal had gone; the mother had been advised that amputation and a prosthetic leg were the only treatment we could offer to get her daughter walking again, and one night she had taken the child and disappeared.

✛

On my last day in Kuito, Rosa lined up some problem cases. She could easily operate on them alone – her surgery experience was fresher than mine, and she had a deftness of touch that carried her through the most demanding of procedures – but I knew what it meant to have a colleague with whom to share the otherwise solitary weight of surgical decision-making; no other field of medicine carries so much individual responsibility. Our most complex operation was on the woman whose burst abdominal wound I'd reclosed. When she'd first arrived at the hospital, hit in the belly by shell fragments, she'd been so malnourished that the healing of her tissues had been affected. The places where her intestines were sutured had broken down and now the bowel leaked through multiple fistulas. Unless these were repaired she would die, of starvation and sepsis. Rosa and I worked together, re-joining the gut and putting in drains before re-closing the abdomen. Her prognosis remained uncertain. When it was time to leave for the airstrip to get my flight, Rosa accompanied me out to the hospital steps. We embraced and she returned to the operating room and her next case. I sought out Jesùs and Eduardo to say farewell, leaving them with small gifts – my stethoscope, my Portuguese-English dictionary – that could never match the wealth of the experiences we'd shared.

The UN aircraft gained height, circling steeply above the skyward-pointing plane wreck and the zigzag trenches at the end of the runway. To the east, where the front ran, pillars of smoke rose as they had done on the day of my arrival. I dozed in my seat until roused by the change in engine note as we throttled down to land in Luanda. Returning to the city was unsettling. Street-corner peddlers sold bootleg DVDs of Hollywood war films. White four-by-four vehicles of two hundred relief organisations formed hooting traffic jams. Aid agency heads of mission and oil company executives complained about the hardship of having their provisions flown in; in this case, imported from Europe and South Africa for the city's luxury dollar-supermarkets. Nobody talked about the legless veterans begging by the roadside, their uniform trousers pinned up over their stumps, or the food transport planes taking off over the city, except to grumble that they destroyed the peace of the beach. The clubs along the palm-fringed *Ilha* – a long spit of sand forming the seaward edge of Luanda Bay – set out their menu prices in dollars and the old *entrepôt* warehouses along the waterfront were being turned into designer bars and discos, playing the latest Western hits. The president's daughter owned the most popular beach bar; government connections were essential in order to obtain licences for these establishments. Portuguese ex-colonists were returning to start businesses and resume their old lifestyle; their yachts rocked at anchor below the terrace restaurant of the Clube Naval de Luanda.

Some days later I was on an airliner travelling from Luanda back to Johannesburg. Drinks were served, and the pilot's voice came over the address system. 'We are going to thirty-seven thousand feet,' he said, 'a little higher than usual. We'll also be flying further west than usual, to avoid the area around the town of Kuito where there is an active military situation. We expect to land in Johannesburg in approximately three and a half hours. Enjoy the flight.'

The land stretched below, jigsaw patches of bush traversed by winding, dried-out watercourses. I looked towards the eastern horizon. The place where Kuito lay was blurred by dust or smoke. I thought about the overflowing surgical wards, the agony of the emergency room, the half-light that filtered through the tent canvas of the critical feeding centre. A few days later I heard that shells were falling on the edge of town and all food flights suspended after a surface-to-air missile exploded near two UN transport planes on their approach to the landing strip. But as far as the rest of the world was concerned, there would still be no crisis in Kuito.

9

Hospital-Acquired Infection

There was something elemental about life in Kuito that I'd been unable to forget: its atmosphere of ruin and survival and last breaths, with each small victory weighed against the war's pitiless folly. I was preparing to return there in February 2002 on another surgical assignment when I heard that Savimbi was dead, shot down when his headquarters column was ambushed by government forces. Guy was in Kuito when the officer credited with firing the fatal burst arrived in town. The young major had been brought that night to the Esplanade Bar, where he'd taken up station in a big armchair (who knew where such a piece of furniture might have been lurking all that time in Kuito) in the centre of the room. In dark glasses, his camouflage battle dress freshly pressed, the man had sat immobile as people filed past to add their tributes, the tables and floor around him filling with bottles of beer and whisky while he remained planted like a sphinx amidst that forest of glass on which the paraffin lamps glinted.

Bereft of the war's sharp realities, left only with that cinematic image, the next deployment I was offered seemed oddly appropriate.

The telephone rang.

'I understand you know about trauma surgery,' said a woman. 'It's Kirstie speaking, from Central Hospital.'

I professed my ignorance of the institution.

'You know, the medical drama? Been running for years, you must know it. We're told it's the most watched programme among hospital doctors, after *ER*.'

'Oh. Of course I must know it. What can I do for you?'

'Well, the story is that Claret-Clyster, the senior surgeon – you know the one, grey hair, posh accent, drink problem – is at home and his brother Steve arrives. Now, Steve's no good, we know that from the last series, and he's using heroin and joined up with these bank robbers and there's been an explosion when they tried to blow the safe and it went wrong and now they've turned up at his house on the run with this wounded robber and they want him to operate.'

There was a silence.

'Are you with me?' asked Kirstie.

I hadn't seen this particular programme, though I could imagine the format. A perennial feature of hospital staff-rooms, alongside the smell of burned toast, was the television set tuned to a hospital drama. Patients – violin prodigies with brain tumours, last-chance-pregnancy fashion models, epileptic airline pilots – were forever being rushed to the operating room by the got-the-shakes surgeon, nymphomaniac nurse and alcoholic anaesthetist amidst a welter of barked TLAs (Three-Letter Acronyms) and the portentous symphony of the machines that go *beep*. I'd always found it hard to suspend disbelief at such melodramatic overload. The sort of emergency triage practised in the austere conditions of war zones, where a blood pressure reading is not always available, relies on a largely intuitive system for the rapid assessment of patients – breathing rate, skin tone, pallor of lips, the restlessness that signifies incipient shock – in order to sort casualties into their priorities for treatment. So a certain cognitive dissonance was inevitable whenever the TV doctors emoted, with much flourishing of the defibrillator paddles, around a case who appeared to be at worst in the 'lightly wounded, can wait' category.

'We need a surgical advisor on location for a couple of days' shooting,' continued Kirstie, 'someone whom the director can consult about how you'd do trauma surgery but not in a hospital. You know, improvising.'

'I see.' I improvised. 'How about in a hairdresser's? You could call the episode "Short Back-and-Insides".'

'Um,' said Kirstie. I sensed that she was wondering about my suitability for the job. 'This is actually about operating with the sort of stuff you'd have in a kitchen. We'll pay you, of course. Is that something you could help us with?'

'Probably. It would be helpful to have an idea what kind of surgery we'll be dealing with,' I said. 'What kind of injury.'

'Hold on.' Over the line came a rustling of pages. 'It says here liver.'

'A bent spoon makes a reasonable retractor,' I offered, gratis.

'Great. That's great!' Kirstie paused to note this down. 'We'll send you a script today. Cheerio.'

The house that the location scouts had chosen for Claret-Clyster's home was set in an exclusive area of London, on the edge of Hampstead Heath. I found it by the mobile dressing rooms parked along the street and the crew-caterer's truck with tea and ginger biscuits standing at the gate. Built in the 1920s in the International Modern style, the building's clean spaces managed to retain their elegance despite the clutter of cables, booms, cameras and lights set up in the kitchen area. The cast were already assembled. The surgeon was in pinstripe suit, about to set off for work when surprised by the gone-wrong bruvva and his criminal consorts, all sporting ne'er-do-well leather jackets. The wounded man lay in the hallway, being ushered into his role by the razoring of his shirt to suggest that he'd been caught in a blast, plus some artful layering of artificial blood.

I stayed out of the way while scenes were shot around the front door: the arrival of the gang, the exchange between their leader and the injured man that hinted at a lovers' bond. The disdainful surgeon and his long-lost brother exchanged bitter lines that would serve viewers as an *aide-memoire* of their fractured relationship. Then the first bit of surgical advice was called for. I suggested that a man with a severely scripted abdominal wound would tend to lie as still as possible, guarding against the agony of movement. The director corrected me swiftly; he had seen enough emergency room dramas to know that the patient would be screaming and threshing about. Then we were ready for a run-through rehearsal of the kitchen scene and all of us from every department and discipline – Camera, Lights, Sound, Makeup, Costume and the rest – were gathered in the room for the initial set-up. The wounded man was carried in, his lover entreating and threatening, while Claret-Clyster turned back his cuffs and the continuity person catalogued every detail in a barrage of Polaroids.

The operation was to be conducted on the kitchen table; a futuristic piece of furniture put together by the set carpenters – perhaps in evocation of the house's architecture – with squares of glass set into its surface so that some of the action could be filmed from beneath. Someone from Props offered me a selection of utensils to use as surgical instruments and I scratched my head over cleavers, corers, spatulas and salad spoons. I found a small sharp knife – the director preferred something much larger – and intimated the impossibility of doing liver surgery without proper forceps and clamps; a real surgeon, I suggested, would simply pack clean cloths into the wound (paper kitchen-roll wouldn't do) and transfer the casualty directly to hospital for resuscitation and treatment. The director looked at me as though I were an utter wimp.

The Prosthetics Department had made an artificial skin of latex that fitted over the body of the wounded actor. Ragged holes had been scorched into the belly with a hot wire to represent the injury that had penetrated the liver, with a fine tube attached near the underside of the lacerations to dribble stage blood through the wound. For the actual operation another false skin stood by, with an incision through it and a pouch on its under-surface representing the abdominal cavity. The script called for major surgery and close-up views of dramatic things going on inside that belly. Prosthetics handed me a bag containing differently coloured and textured bits of rubber from which I was invited to select my organs. I rummaged about for a liver, a gallbladder and a length of bowel.

'During surgery that's all going to be held out of the way,' said the organ donor authoritatively, 'with a bent spoon.'

But human anatomy, which requires the colon to be retracted downwards during liver surgery, had been stood on its head. The false belly had its inner space extending upwards from the incision.

'Maybe we could turn it round,' proposed Prosthetics.

This move would place the incision on the wrong side of the abdomen, with the nipples over the groins. We tried it this way and that until the shout of 'Ready' went up, when we shrugged, settled the latex sheet on the actor, anointed it with blood and were batted outside by the clipboard of the production manager.

During filming only the cast and cinematographers remained in the kitchen. From the pantry, a sound-man extended his overhead boom. The rest of us joined the director on canvas chairs set out on the lawn, our distance from his viewing screen a yardstick of our importance in the production. The cameras rolled and I realised I was witnessing a master at work. The director knew in advance every angle he'd need. He set up the shots briskly, asking me after each one if there had been any technical errors or incongruities in the take and then moving on. As we watched the sequence of two-shots, reverses, cut-aways and close-ups in the monitor's tight frame, I was seduced by artifice. The wrist-twist that I'd shown the surgeon in order to get his hand in under the rib-cage looked exactly as awkward as it is in reality, and seeing the pasta tongs slip from his blood-slick fingers I found myself wanting to elbow aside the sound technician's boom and get into the belly with some proper instruments.

The whole experience was a joy: the badinage among the gaffers with their belt-rolls of coloured tape, the lighting men's acerbic wit and the fastidious professionalism of the supporting specialists. Props looked after the amount of blood on the furniture, laying it on with a tiny spoon more suited to cocaine until they were encouraged to splash it about a bit. Blood on a latex belly was the responsibility of Prosthetics, but any appearing on an actor's clothes was applied by Costumes. Facial gore was looked after by Makeup. Overlaps between the disciplines resulted in little contretemps, usually good-humoured and readily resolved. Life on set was rather like working in a hospital, and I was delighted that the series continued to make use of me when the story line dealt with unconventional surgical crises.

Scripts would arrive in the mail a couple of days in advance. I found the plot and characterisation pleasingly complex – good doctor versus bad doctor, medical success or disaster, sex, love, addiction and betrayal – carried through a half-dozen interwoven story lines that addressed issues of moral judgement and social diversity and even the existential proposition that death might be something that gave our lives meaning. I'd read, entranced, on the ride to the studios, taking an early morning train running empty out of London towards the west. The service travelled through leafy suburbs and meadows that always seemed to be splashed with sunlight, stopping at stations with names suggesting an urbane gentility. Then it plunged under a long, forested ridge through a tunnel that after ten minutes of rattling darkness delivered me at the other end to the film-set and the world of medical make-believe.

Scene: operating theatre. Domineering consultant and sensitive subordinate are at the sink, scrubbing their hands for surgery. As the taps are turned off – figuratively, for they have never been on; running water makes too much noise on the soundtrack – the consultant takes his junior to task about displaying excessive ethical scrupulousness. Through the conversation they are drying their hands, putting on surgical gowns, donning gloves. The combination of nuanced dialogue and complex action means that there are errors in the actors' delivery and several retakes are necessary. Each time new sterile gown packs are opened, fresh gloves unsealed and the bin in the corridor fills with debris at two hundred pounds a go. I think of how handy this stuff would have been in places where we operated with gloves that were washed and hung in the sun to dry before reuse. The director's concern is that the impact of the lines is being lost because the actors' surgical masks hide their expressions.

'I want the scene shot without masks,' he announces. 'They can put them on afterwards.'

I explain that touching the masks would render the surgeons' hands unsterile.

'We'll let a nurse tie them on,' he declares, but after a comedy of masks being positioned over eyes or under chins this plan is abandoned and the action left as it is. One of the actors winks at me.

'I depend on that mask,' he murmurs. 'It's hard to deliver this mixture of bathos and bollocks with a straight face.'

The tower block in which the hospital drama was filmed had the precise aesthetic of a National Health Service hospital. Floors were fitted out as wards and X-ray units, with authentic posters along the corridors featuring talking bacteria or warning of penalties for assaults on staff. The linoleum had exactly the right shade of throat-lozenge green. The operating theatres were fully fitted out, except that I'd never seen such equipment in the many NHS hospitals at which I'd worked. There were trays of new instruments of the finest quality, the jaws of clamps and scissors meeting crisply. Surgical tables, anaesthetic machines, closed-circuit operating video cameras and theatre lights were all state-of-the-art, of a standard that I might never otherwise have believed existed if I hadn't seen them in real life on the film-set.

The operations themselves were very wondrous events. One major case was a character whom the scriptwriter had flung from his motorcycle onto iron railings, one of which had penetrated deep into his abdomen. In the previous scene the fire service had sawed through the spike and brought the casualty straight to hospital, where he now hovered in theatrical *extremis* while the anaesthetist prepared him for surgery. The ventilator sighed, the coloured lines on the monitor wriggled. The actor playing the patient lay on the operating table with fake drips in his arms and an endotracheal tube, cut short, clamped between his teeth. Green drapes bordered the prosthesis on his belly, from which jutted a length of realistic-looking black iron rod. A Props person switched on the wall-mounted viewing screen and slapped up an X-ray. It showed a standard abdominal view – the white outline of pelvis, vertebrae and ribs, the shadows of gas and fluid in the bowel – and, pointing into the vitals, the black, spear-shaped outline of the railing.

'I think,' I suggested, 'that the railing should be white.'

Props was tolerant, despite the fact that I was trespassing on his territory.

'No, mate. You do get white railings, I grant you, but black ones are commoner. So I made the thing black.'

I tried to explain that X-rays didn't work like that. He remained forgiving.

'X-ray's a sort of photo, right? Bones are white, because they're white. Railing's black' – the man pointed at the rod – ''cos it's black.'

There was a debate into which people from all the disciplines on set were drawn, while the patient-actor sweltered under his layers of rubber. Someone went off to find the child-that-swallowed-the-ambulance-keys X-ray featured in a previous episode, and it was put up on the screen for comparison. The keys were white. We tried to modify the X-ray plate by sticking paper over the railing's outline, but the black spear had actually looked considerably more impressive. Eventually we left it on the screen with the light off, as an unilluminated blur in the background.

The actors entered to take their marks. I'd always found them utterly convincing in their roles; the man who played the chief anaesthetist was someone I'd allow to put me to sleep anytime, and the surgeons delivered their lines with appropriate professionalism. The surgeon was supposed to swab the protruding rod with disinfectant, while asking his registrar whether she'd ever had an impaling. She was capable of expressing an extraordinary range of emotions with her eyes, which here flashed a riposte above her face mask. Then he was to seize the end of the metal with both hands and pull it from the wound, before requesting a scalpel to 'get in and see what we've got'. The dramatic impact was obvious, but again a nagging realism intervened: I was too aware of the structures and organs that would have been transfixed in such an injury. Reluctantly, I suggested that it would be better to open the belly with the spike still in place, so that one could be ready, for example, with an arterial clamp to prevent a major haemorrhage as the point was removed. After more conversation between the departments, a script revision was made and the operation carried through to its uplifting conclusion.

✪

Real clinical situations could be surreal enough to try the most creative of scriptwriters. Sometimes, to pay my rent and subsidise my volunteer surgical assignments, I took weekend work in private hospitals as a resident medical officer. The food was excellent – these exclusive institutions engaged professional chefs – but they were not such good places to be unwell. Unlike acute NHS hospitals, with dedicated 'crash' teams of doctors and nurses on call for emergencies, survival rates of cardiac arrest here were lower and could be complicated by unforeseen factors. During one resuscitation the anaesthetist and I were much hampered by shrieking relatives, who kept bursting into the room to throw themselves across the patient's body. Sister and staff-nurse held them back to prevent electrocution while we ripped open the man's pyjamas in order to apply the defibrillator. Lamentations redoubled as packs of banknotes tumbled out.

At other times I worked in private clinics, performing health screening examinations. Generally this was a service for the 'worried well', their complaints at the cosmetic end of the health and beauty spectrum. Most had company medical plans or comprehensive health insurance and believed the advertisements of the private health providers who promised 'to make your body our business'. The medical consultations were recorded on computerised templates, ticking boxes and activating drag-down menus that allowed the marketing executives to graph both the Uptake of Product and our individual productivity. Clients would be welcomed by the rich teal carpet (chosen to suggest an ambience informal yet professional), the flower arrangements and the seamless delivery of the smart receptionist; all reassuring them that they'd get their money's worth and that private medicine would take away their problems. In the waiting room they sat down with a glass of fruit-juice and a muesli bar to tackle the questionnaire with its urbane interrogation: How many times a week do you have business lunches: Once? Twice? Daily?

There were patients for whom these consultations were ideal: the big-bellied potentates with their multinational business and well-travelled hypochondriasis; the internist in Paris, the cardiologist in Toronto, the allergist in New York and the fill-in medicals when they passed through London in case the others had missed something. They'd list mysterious, inexplicable symptoms in unrelated body systems, trumping each attempt at diagnosis with a new complaint and demanding referrals to multiple specialists. Attempts to offer basic health advice – eat less fat, stop smoking, take more exercise – were poorly received; what right had I, a paid servant, to criticise their lifestyles? I had finished examining one man's abdomen when its owner seized my hand and pressed it down again into the rolls of fat.

'Do that more,' he ordered. I explained that the examination was complete.

'I feel it is good for me,' he said. 'I need a doctor who will do this when I require it. I will speak to your employers about taking over your contract.'

There were also the very, very worried well who demanded 'the test that guarantees that I don't have cancer', refusing to accept my explanation that this very general term referred to a myriad of different diseases affecting every body tissue in a different way, and that no single investigation would detect all its forms. A couple of times I told an insistent patient that the only absolute confirmation that cancer was not present would be to dissect his body into its constituent cells and pass each one under a microscope; the pathologist's report would be the closest thing to a guarantee, but it would of course be posthumous. At least one reached for his wallet and wanted to know the cost. But usually the joke collapsed: these customers expected the assurance that their money could buy them immunity from death. I suspected they were accustomed to a type of society doctor, at home in plush parlours and drawing rooms, who colluded in these fantasies.

I found drawing rooms a much tougher arena. My recreational drinking at parties would be interrupted by people who'd discovered I was a doctor. Most were simply angling for a free consultation, but a few guests relished the opportunity to work through personal issues regarding the profession. They'd recount one of two basic stories – both illustrating the criminal ineptness of doctors – that had invariably genuinely actually happened to an almost-acquaintance.

The first was the missed diagnosis: 'The cousin of a woman who takes her cat to the same vet as my mum, right, well her father-in-law went to see his general practitioner with backache and the GP said it was arthritis but it was cancer of the back and two months later he was dead.'

The other version additionally confirmed doctors' cruelty and backwardness: 'My girlfriend's aunt's hairdresser's stepmother,' a middle-aged children's writer informed me, 'was diagnosed with leukaemia and told that she had to have chemotherapy. They gave her twelve weeks to live. Instead she went to a natural healer and six months later she's absolutely fine.'

I expressed the hope that she was indeed fine, and tried to explain how unlikely it was that the woman would have been given a prognosis of such shattering precision; the most aggressive cancers kill around ninety-five percent of sufferers within five years of diagnosis, but that means that five percent will be still alive, so doctors avoid committing themselves to rigid predictions of life-expectancy. The man remained unmollified, so I tried an old joke.

'It's true there was this doctor, gave this bloke six months to live. At the end of that time the man hadn't paid him, so he gave him another six months.'

'I don't think this is anything to snicker about,' snapped the writer, but a passing alternative therapist, who hadn't heard the joke before, laughed generously. Confident that I supported complementary medicine – for what intelligent doctor wouldn't, in these post-rational times? – she gave me her card in order that I might refer my patients to her group of naturopathic practitioners for a revolutionary treatment they were developing.

'The thing is to identify the new thing: timeless yet effective, like the Hopi Ear Candle. Take colonic irrigation.' She hopped into the writer's vacated place on the sofa. 'Take crystal healing. Two well-established forms of therapy; everyone's heard of them. So our idea is simple: to combine the power of both. It's called colonic crystals.'

'You mean –'

'Yes.' She lifted one buttock from her seat and made a holistic, inserting movement with her forefinger. 'It sets the healing power of crystal rays to work inside you.'

✺

I took a real job, as a surgeon in a National Health Service hospital on the edge of London. The operating department had high windows from which I could look out over the city as I scrubbed my hands before surgery. Great blue clouds sailed up the Thames estuary, once Britain's gateway to its overseas Empire. On the horizon, where London's docks had stood, the towers of the Canary Wharf financial district glittered like a growth of crystals. My older patients had seen the area burn under German bombs. Some had served in the avenging armies. Others had arrived from the old colonies: India, Africa, the Caribbean. After the war they'd been the builders of economic reconstruction and then watched the industries decline. Some of their children now worked in those distant, shining towers, or were 'on the disability', reconciled to unemployment. Some of their grandchildren were among the pregnant teenage girls sitting outside the maternity block, puffing on cigarettes as they waited to deliver the next generation.

My involvement in the lives of these people was limited – long enough to examine them, assess them for operation and through my surgical efforts hopefully to make their physical lives better – but through this brief intimacy I was aware of deeper stories, of adversity and triumph, sadness and single motherhood and fulfilled love, just like the patients of Central Hospital. This bunch, though, were much more entertaining.

'Trouble peeing, Doc,' they'd tell me, 'it's me prostitute gland.'

I was called to the ward to see a ninety-year-old dear who was unable to walk.

'How long have you been bedridden?' I asked her.

'Oo, not for years, Doctor,' she cackled.

Even my colleagues lacked reverence. One afternoon the emergency department was on standby for the end of a football game between two London teams whose supporters were known for their post-match violence; already the first split heads had arrived, full of beery belligerence. While the Casualty doctors were thus occupied, the waiting room had filled suddenly with a mass of retired persons that occupied every seat, as well as the fleet of wheelchairs normally kept folded in a storeroom beside the porter's lodge. An ambulance stretcher-crew was battling to wheel a bloodied football partisan through the throng when the Emergency consultant appeared.

He turned to the reception nurse. 'Who are all these people?'

'A pensioners' outing,' she explained. 'Their coach was involved in a little accident, so the driver brought them here. In case they might need treatment for shock.'

'Shock?' The consultant's voice rose. 'Shock as in a major drop in blood pressure? Shock requiring resuscitation to prevent organ failure and death?' He looked around at the grey-heads, some of whom, making themselves comfortable, had unwrapped sandwiches.

'All those of you suffering from shock, stand up,' he ordered. The majority of his audience rose to their feet, though some needed a moment or two to re-cap their thermoses.

'Well, you lot can piss off, for a start,' the consultant declared, to good-natured grumbling.

The radio in the operating theatre was tuned usually to a local station, giving news and travel reports and advertising the unmissable offers down the High Street. The people here were a community; patients, nurses and doctors lived in the area. They liked their local NHS hospital, even if the operating theatres were last fitted out twenty years before and the oldest ward blocks had been built originally as a prison barracks for Italian soldiers captured in the North African desert. One of my patients, a child during the war, described taking a detour each morning on his way to school in order to throw insults at the POWs being marched to work in the fields. His voice, to my surprise, still carried a boyhood loathing. I told him my father's story of the day Italy had surrendered in September 1943. An Italian prison camp had stood near his field hospital. Most of the inmates were jubilant, but an enraged fascist had armed himself with a plank bearing at its end a six-inch nail, with which he rampaged through the camp smacking his celebrating countrymen in the belly. My father had spent the night in surgery repairing punctured stomachs and intestines.

My patient looked uneasy. 'We were always being told how they were the enemy,' he said, 'but I suppose they were just ordinary blokes.' He gave an embarrassed laugh. 'In wartime they get you to swallow all kinds of rubbish.'

But it wasn't only in wartime, for the politicians had recently published their National Health Service Improvement Plan, which promised to modernise health-care provision through market efficiency. A few miles away, a grove of construction cranes marked the site of a much-trumpeted super-hospital that would replace all the region's existing facilities. Being built under the terms of the government's Private Finance Initiative – at considerable cost to the Health Service, which would pay commercial rent to the private sector builders – the new hospital would provide fewer beds but significant on-site retail space. Any treatment shortfall would be taken up by private surgical centres run by very-much-for-profit healthcare consortia, that would also take over the hospital's laboratory, X-ray, kitchen and laundry services. The modernising minister running the Department of Health had also designed the new contracts being pressed on doctors. I'd attended a lecture for general practitioners on the way their professional obligations were now to be defined.

'The contract is based on a "quality and outcomes" framework,' the GPs were informed. 'Clinical practice has ten domains producing a hundred and forty-six evidence-based indicators worth five hundred and fifty points. The Practice Factor is calculated by dividing the square root of practice prevalence by the square root of national prevalence. This is used to establish a practice's performance-based operating budget. An average practice list of five thousand eight hundred patients earns seventy-five pounds a point. . . .' The new contract for hospital consultants was equally tricky. We'd be expected to renounce the right to base treatment decisions on clinical judgement. Instead, a management 'business plan' would dictate the hours we'd work and which patients we treated – in response to the government's electioneering promises to bring down hospital waiting times, rather than according to medical urgency – for which surgeons should be prepared to perform extra operating sessions at night or on weekends.

Doctors were generally well regarded by the public – polls consistently showed their 'trust rating' at over ninety percent – and their professional objections that these priority shifts would damage patient care were upsetting to the politicians, who held the ranking of 'most mistrusted'. The government had been relieved, therefore, when the case emerged of a psychopathic GP who over the years had managed to murder some 150 of his patients, just about the time that a scandal broke about a paediatric cardiac surgery unit, performing highly complex operations on exceedingly unwell babies, that had an unacceptable run of post-operative deaths. Headlines sprouted in the tabloid press, fertilised by unattributable sources, implying that far from helping the public, medical practitioners neglected their National Health Service commitments in favour of perfecting their golf swings and pandering to private patients; apart, that is, from the doctors who were negligent butchers or serial killers. Psychometric profiling was proposed to expose our criminal tendencies, along with 'virtual chaperones' – video cameras recording every aspect of the clinical process – for patient protection.

This manufactured hysteria had a precedent of sorts. During the Doctors' Plot, Stalin's final set of show trials in 1953, the Russian medical profession was accused, among other crimes, of killing patients as part of a counter-revolutionary plan to discredit the Kremlin and undermine its cosmic advances in Soviet medicine. The newspaper *Tass* vociferated against 'these enemies of the people, who ... by taking advantage of their status as physicians and abusing the trust of their patients, deliberately ignored the data of objective examinations, made incorrect diagnoses and thus brought about the death of their charges'. Editorials demanded execution, which was accordingly administered to a number of 'ringleaders'; many other doctors were sentenced to the gulags for long periods of self-criticism and re-education.

Of course, no death sentence faced us, simply the introduction of a compulsory annual revalidation folder to assess our continuing competence to practice (although there'd never been any suggestion that the killer GP had been medically incompetent, just insane). The paperwork included showing proof of how we were addressing patient complaints in ways that would improve our clinical practice. A colleague told me how, at his last revalidation, he had explained to the evaluator that he could not fulfil this part of the assessment because there'd been no complaints made against him.

'No complaints?' The assessor had looked solemn. 'That's not going to look good. How are you going to identify your Core Competency performance goals to meet and improve on?'

Exposure of malfeasance had permeated the Health Service bureaucracy. On my second day in my hospital job, about to commence the seventh case on my operating list, I'd been interrupted by the opening of the theatre door. A woman leaned in, who I noticed was not wearing surgical greens.

'Excuse me,' she said firmly, 'but I'm afraid you have to stop operating.'

'Why? What's going on?'

'An administrative matter. Could I talk to you outside, please?'

Shedding my gloves, I went out to the corridor. The woman, in a smart business suit, was waiting in the sister's office. I noticed that her high heels had stabbed straight through the sterile shoe-covers provided for visitors to the operating department.

'I'm from Clinical Resources Management,' she announced, 'and a problem has come to our attention. Occupational Health Management has identified the report you submitted regarding your hepatitis immunity as not coming from our hospital laboratory.'

'That's true. Three months ago, when you offered me this job, you required me to provide proof of my hepatitis status. I had it done at the clinic where I was working at the time, and you've had the report since then. What's wrong with it?'

'I'm not saying you'd be guilty of medical dishonesty' – she gave a sort of ventriloquist's laugh that spared her lips – 'but you could have presented a false report by using someone else's blood. I've got a doctor right here to get a fresh sample, that I can certify I witnessed being taken from you.'

She beckoned in an embarrassed-looking anaesthetist, who wrapped a tourniquet around my arm and stuck in a needle.

'It'll take a few hours to get that result from your lab,' I said as the blood tube filled, 'so perhaps you could apply your management abilities to cancelling the rest of my surgical cases for the day, and explaining to the patients why I can't operate on them this afternoon.'

'But you have to operate,' she squeaked, 'Waiting list reduction is a Key Performance Indicator!'

'If I couldn't operate five minutes ago because you didn't have acceptable proof of my hepatitis immunity, I can hardly operate now.'

'Oh, but you can,' she said confidently. 'I'll state that it's necessary, on Clinical Management authority.'

The NHS Improvement Plan was evident in large matters – a cut in hospital beds, so that the remaining ones were occupied without let-up – and small ones – hospitals no longer had their own cleaners, the tender having gone to the contractor that would do the job for the lowest price. Often this did not include cleaning caked blood from the white rubber operating boots worn by surgeons. A coincident explosion in hospital-acquired infection had been addressed by creating a high-profile, government-appointed 'Infection Tsar', whose executive team dreamed up the talking bacteria posters. But the government's next New Idea – publishing performance tables of treatment outcomes – revealed a lurking catastrophe: near-on fifty percent of hospitals, surgeons and other specialists were below average. The government knew that its re-election might hang on the public impression of health standards, and a solution was quickly thought up: Patient Choice. Everyone, promised the prime minister, would be offered the right to treatment by the specialist and hospital of their preference. One visionary Department of Health official even foresaw oncology patients prescribing their own chemotherapy. Indeed, the very term 'patient' would soon be outmoded; we were advised to think, rather, of 'health consumers'.

Doctors reported that patients, given the choice – 99.3 percent in a recent study – wanted treatment, without infection, at their local hospital. Other clinicians complained about the bureaucracy of organising referrals to centres across the country and the costly new 'choice-facilitation' managers needed to administer the plan. It was clear at once to the politicians that these quibbling doctors were part of the problem, defenders of outdated practices that prevented the Improved NHS achieving its new potential. Re-education would be provided for all. It was hoped this would raise standards across the board, so that eventually ninety-five or even one hundred percent of clinicians would be above average. A notice board in the operating department sitting room listed 'development days' to be attended by its staff. These were run by commercial companies contracted 'to meet health-care learning needs', by providing courses for doctors and nurses in professional goal visualisation. Other consultancies performed 'empathy audits' to identify those requiring training in caring, communication and warmth-building. The effect on waiting lists – when surgery was replaced by re-training sessions – would be addressed by using funds from the health budget for operation-cancellation-reduction managers and rapid discharge co-ordinators to further speed up bed turnover and improve business efficiency.

Sceptical doctors continued to wonder whether this money might have been better directed towards increasing the number of hospital beds or cleaning those surgical boots. But the time for talk, the politicians told us, was past; now it was time for action. They were progressive and dynamic and busy on their next campaign, the World Improvement Plan. Non-conforming 'rogue' states that failed to embrace Freedom would be forcibly introduced to the benefits of Democracy and the Global Market. Those of us who professed doubt about this crusade were simply ignorant of the overwhelming intelligence data accessible to our leaders regarding the mortal menaces that could be launched against us in a matter of minutes. We should all be very frightened. The operating room radio interspersed their broadcasts with advertisements for private health care.

'Don't play Russian Roulette with your life,' they barked. 'Get those haemorrhoids fixed NOW!'

10

Fragmentation Wounds

From somewhere in the clinic's courtyard came a bellow of rage. The office was crowded with men who stood against the walls while the director and I talked. Some of them had been guarding the compound gate when we'd arrived and had let us in grudgingly, fingers on the triggers of their weapons that were pointed to the sky. The voice outside roared with fury and a body hurled itself against the door; the metal panels, battered by looters, warped ominously. My colleagues – two women doctors from the Iraqi Ministry of Health – paled under their headscarves. The guards exchanged glances but their beards made it difficult to read their expressions. No-one moved. Another crash and the door shrieked and sprang from its frame. A fist came through the gap; above it a face. The man's eyes caught mine, bulging and apoplectic. The mullah's soldiers decided evidently that the point had been made. Two of them shouldered the man back and the bent door was pushed to. The clinic director's smile had gone and his pleasant features looked creased and discomforted.

'We have no drugs, no water,' he said. 'There is a lot of sickness. The people here are very angry. They say that everything in Baghdad has been destroyed on purpose.'

The director saw us out into the courtyard. As we emerged, our driver threw down his cigarette and opened the vehicle's doors, calling urgently.

'We must go at once,' said motherly Dr Saria. 'There is shooting nearby. He says it is not safe.'

Turbaned militiamen threw open the iron gate and we bumped out into the street. A burned-out ambulance stood at the curb. The iron railings of the goods yards opposite were hung with black banners carrying cursive Arabic: the names and circumstances of those who had died in this neighbourhood of the city. The black flags formed an unbroken line all the way down the street.

'Pathology,' wrote the visionary nineteenth century German histologist Rudolf Virchow, 'is politics writ large.' Nowhere was this assertion more true than in Baghdad, where I'd arrived in April 2003 shortly after US forces had taken the city. Coalition forces had bombed Baghdad for nineteen days, and though they claimed that only military resources were targeted, it was clear that there had been many civilian casualties. Then, during their advance in to the city from the west and south, the US forces had used the tactic called 'reconnaissance by fire'; the video clips had shown, as well as burning tanks (the same short sequence of them, hull-down in the ditches gouting smoke), the family cars with figures slumped at the wheel or huddled in the foot-wells.

Now, two weeks after the Americans had declared Baghdad conquered, the deaths continued. Gunfire crackled, sometimes distant, usually just outside on the street. Buildings blazed across the skyline. Each night the American position at the nearby university campus came under attack and from the hotel roof we could see the tracers fly; red streaks passed just over our heads and whacked into the building behind. Army units were jumpy and uncertain and ready to open up on anything they didn't understand. Too often their targets were civilians, and cavalcades of cars, loaded with the injured and the dead, arrived at hospitals that – despite the obligation of the Occupying Force to provide essential services – were scarcely functioning.

I was here as a volunteer surgeon, but operating was difficult. The city's hospitals had treated many wounded during the bombing, depleting emergency stores. Following the arrival of the Americans, much of the remainder had been looted, the pillage continuing even as staff tried to deal with arriving casualties. Operating rooms resembled charnel-houses, with discarded surgeons' gloves, crusted dressings and bloody clothes caked underfoot. Until the mid-1980s Iraq had boasted the most advanced health care in the Middle East; now the buildings appeared derelict, their dusty windows broken by blast or criss-crossed with tape against fragmentation. Fuel shortages meant the generators could at best light only small areas of the hospitals and were unable to power the elevators; injured were carried up the stairs to the operating tables, their wounds jetting. Water arrived in buckets, instruments could not be sterilised. Under these conditions the Iraqi surgeons – experienced, often with specialist qualifications obtained in England or the US – were operating only when it was entirely unavoidable, because of the risk of sepsis. I'd helped with some emergency cases, but most problems could not be solved with surgical skills.

The young Iraqi doctors working as volunteers in the emergency rooms were concerned about our safety. As the afternoons advanced, the treatment areas became deserted of staff, until by darkness the buildings had been abandoned to gangs of AK-47–carrying looters and to patients, defended on the wards by their gun-wielding relatives to stop the beds themselves being taken and sold. Shooting surged and ebbed until the morning when the medical staff would to start patching the casualties that had been dumped at the entrance through the night, while the local mosque saw to the bodies of those that had bled to death where they lay.

✪

In planning for the war, all the international medical relief organisations had expected that surgeons would be essential. From November 2002, four months before the first air-strikes, I had been in contact with aid groups with whom I'd worked previously. They were interested in my surgical experience in northern Iraq during the Kurdish uprising that followed the last Gulf War – and in my South African passport, which might offer me easier access to the country than would be possible for citizens of the Coalition nations – but no-one seemed certain what sort of medical intervention would be required. Some organisations planned camps and field hospitals to receive refugees from the towns, the sort of crisis we'd seen in Kurdistan. Others foresaw the population staying in the urban centres, which might become battlegrounds as Coalition forces fought street by street with the Iraqi army; US units were reportedly being trained by Israeli instructors in warfare methods used in Palestinian towns. It seemed that the Pentagon intended to direct every aspect of Operation Iraqi Liberation (an early White House appellation, hastily revised when someone in the State Department read the initials), including the humanitarian response.

We heard that American PVOs (private voluntary organisations) were being briefed by Defence officials for a humanitarian intervention that would be unlike any other in history. Their personnel would be positioned in readiness along the Kuwait border. As the invasion rolled forward, their aid teams would be signalled to move to pre-arranged coordinates inside Iraq and set up facilities to receive specified numbers of civilians. These would be herded out of population centres by judicious cruise-missile strikes on the edges of towns that would demarcate a corridor for flight, directing them towards the waiting humanitarian facilities. Once the Iraqi military units remaining in the cities had been obliterated by targeted firepower, the civilian populations would return home. It was anticipated that stability and services would be rapidly re-established by a combination of the Pentagon-directed PVOs and Coalition forces. Independent aid organisations – particularly European ones – were not envisaged as having a role.

Their alternative was to get into Iraq before the war started, by applying to the Iraqi government for permission to operate in their country. This involved submitting a mission proposal to the Iraqi Foreign Ministry with the résumés of personnel who would staff it. The ministry bureaucrats were slow, fearful of spies. One aid group put my name forward but then pondered withdrawing it because I had worked in English hospitals. Another warned me periodically to expect a departure call 'in two days, maybe one'; each time it didn't come I'd phone their office, to be put through to some new staffer who would listen to my explanation that I was the South African surgeon waiting to go to Iraq and request excitedly that I submit my résumé for urgent consideration. A third group discussed a possible mission in Kurdistan. Meanwhile, I watched the countdown with a fearful excitement, my boots, stethoscope and survival kit packed, knowing that those few, agile medical organisations who managed to get their personnel into Baghdad at this stage would have no way of extricating them or sending relief once the first explosions came. At night I'd lie awake in a sweat of claustrophobic terror at the thought of being trapped underground while missiles rained down above. Every time the telephone rang my heart raced.

Then the air war started, reported first-hand by excited journalists from the terrace of their Baghdad hotel. I found myself thinking of my mother's childhood story of the day the Second World War began: the family sitting around the wireless in their village outside Pretoria listening to the news from distant Europe, her older brothers – one just graduated from medical school, the other studying engineering – talking about joining up, and how excited she'd been, convinced that the world had changed forever and there'd be no school tomorrow. I felt a similar expectation as I watched on television the green fireflies of anti-aircraft tracer lofting through the night above Baghdad. Each evening the bombing intensified and I learned the outlines of certain buildings across the Tigris, seen first in silhouette against the pulsing horizon and then side-lit by closer and closer explosions until they themselves became targets. These were described as military assets – telephone exchanges, palaces, government ministries – and their destruction as a precise programme to 'degrade enemy command and communications capability'. There was something prurient in the way the politicians mouthed these morsels of tactical terminology, like thick chocolate. Al-Jezeera Arabic television showed the effects of missile strikes on civilian areas; sometimes the international media would be taken to a scene of carnage where families wept. Our potato-head Minister of Defence blustered about 'selective reporting' and 'giving comfort to the enemy', but I could smell the acrid smoke that clung to the bodies of the wounded as though I were there right now, working in a hospital where the lights flickered and cavalcades of cars pulled up at the entrance leaking blood.

The ground campaign brought an escalation in the verbal mendacity. Coalition forces armed with the world's most advanced weaponry took objective after objective, Iraqi units melting away before them, while the 'embedded' journalists reported skirmishes as great victories and missed the portent of those conquests that required re-pacification for days longer than expected as small Iraqi groups fought back with assault rifles and rocket-propelled grenades. With US forces closing in on Baghdad, aid personnel were being readied to be sent in to relieve the volunteer medical teams that had been helping in the city's hospitals. 'Stand-by' calls came daily from the aid groups. I knew that I'd be going off to serve, with whichever of them was quickest off the mark.

Victory was declared by television – Saddam's toppled statue being revealed to have been supported only by a pair of spindly pipes, analogous perhaps to the ramshackle core of his regime – yet the Iraqi people seemed inexplicably ungrateful to their liberators. The Baghdad square where the statue had stood became the focus of daily demonstrations against the US occupation. All around, the city convulsed and burned and has never since been stilled. I clinched my pack more tightly – the better to run – and clipped to the zip-pull of my jacket a tiny Buddha, given to me in Burma as protection against bullets. At that moment, as though to affirm my rootlessness, an eviction letter arrived. My landlady had vexed my short stay in her property by demanding periodically that I was to leave and then dropping the matter when I requested the legal period of notice. This time, though, her letter was unassailable. Over the phone I explained my imminent departure for Iraq to treat war casualties, with insufficient time to find new accommodation before I left. Her voice became sharp.

'You think your life is *so* important. Well, I have a life too, and I've decided to move you out so I can put the flat on the market. You don't *have* to go to Iraq now, you could just refuse.'

It was almost impossible to answer her. My life's importance was unmeasureable by status or property; it was in the precariousness of situations like Iraq that it acquired definition, became real. I asked whether she'd consider extending the notice period to allow me the chance to move out when I returned. She refused, but in truth I hardly cared. One of the agencies had given me a departure date; I was on my way.

Somehow, even the uncertainty of my mission seemed appropriate. I'd been engaged as a surgeon, but no-one was sure what I would be doing when I got there. A two-man vanguard from the organisation had just arrived in Baghdad to begin an emergency evaluation of the capital's medical facilities, and I might be required to assist in that assessment, or to examine the health situation in

Iraqi Kurdistan where I had worked previously. At the same time, unceasing gunfire on the TV news spoke of surgeons being needed. Much of the material accompanying me and a Canadian colleague from the aid group consisted of communications equipment: satellite phones, modems and Internet software. Instead of flak-jackets we carried three heavy laptop computers for report-writing, crucial to the modern humanitarian mission. I would have to be versatile and adaptable, and mindful of the market pressures at work even in the not-for-profit aid industry: donors want to be associated with high-profile projects, while the competition for public attention means that every agency has to maximise its opportunities for fund-raising. I read through my briefing file on the flight to Amman. It included directions on how to face journalists, how to comport myself before the cameras and what phrases were to be used when talking about the organisation's work.

Rain fell on the Jordanian capital through a chilly grey-yellow light that gleamed off the stone of the apartment blocks. Our Amman-based field director welcomed us with news of sandstorms in Baghdad, and a dense itinerary of briefings and meetings to attend. I shivered in my desert clothes. At a session of UN planners, waiting to be allowed back into Iraq, we learned how humanitarian disasters with a high media profile invariably attract public donations of inappropriate or unusable material; in the Kosovo crisis this had amounted to eighty percent – mainly clothing and food – that had cost the UN millions to store and eventually dump. A lecture on International Humanitarian Law set out the complexities of aid agency relationships with the Occupying Power. If this was failing in its obligations – to provide health care, water, power and security – an aid group could legitimately step in to fulfil those requirements while maintaining its operational independence. Anyone, though, who simply turned up in Baghdad with a load of material and handed it out through official channels was acting as an 'implementing partner' of the military and could not object if they acquired a US army escort and flag atop their trucks.

Agencies from around the world were in town: Emergency Life Support, Operation Mercy, the Mercy Corps, the International Medical Corps, the International Rescue Committee, Rescue Net

International, Northwest Medical Teams International, Medical Aid International, Direct Relief International, Relief International, Relief, Catholic Relief Services, Care, Caritas, Christian Aid, Samaritan's Purse International, the Mennonite Central Committee, the Movement for Peace, Democracy and Freedom, Medics for Vietnam and Peace, Doctors of the World, World Vision and many others. Some handed out press releases about their intentions in Iraq. The American organisations in particular were in love with their own virtue and the moral rightness of their mission. Most were funded though their government's Agency for International Development and directed by ORHA, the Pentagon's Office for Rehabilitation and Humanitarian Assistance, or had been signed up directly by Bechtel, the US corporation disbursing contracts for the reconstruction of Iraq. Of the eighty or so aid groups waiting in Amman, about fifty were American and some half of those defined themselves as Christian organisations, many with an evangelist bent. It seemed that the religious right that had supported Bush's presidency was now being rewarded with a ticket to proselytise in Iraq.

Our group faced more earthly problems. Satellite-phone conversations with our two colleagues already in Baghdad described gunfights for control of hospitals as doctors fought looters trying to strip the pharmacies. The few international agencies in the city were handing out their medical stocks as quickly as possible, for their depots too were targets. Getting to the Iraqi capital was possible only by convoy along the desert highway. Its last hundred miles passed through an area notorious for 'banditry'; the Sunni area around Ar-Ramadi and Falluja whose fiercely independent tribes had never submitted to Saddam's domination and were now holding up trucks from the aid organisations and relieving staff of their satellite phones, matériel and possessions.

'Are you frightened of going to Baghdad?' the field director kept asking. 'You should be frightened.'

But the Canadian and I had made our last calls home; our French logistician, a veteran of aid missions in Angola and Congo, had prepared the equipment, medical supplies and fuel; and the three of us would be joining the next convoy, leaving that night.

The vehicles were required to form up at two A.M. The convoy's organiser was ECHO, the European Community Humanitarian Office, and they were late to arrive. I stood in the street, stamping my feet against the chill. In a doorway sat a pretty girl with her friend, both drunk and giggling, drinking wine from a bottle and not feeling the cold. She wore a little dress and held by their straps little shoes with kitten heels, and she looked so lovely that I wished that I could stay around to discover the Amman party scene and dance with that girl in her impracticably thin dress. Trucks were starting their engines, being marshalled into position by a spiky little Belgian with a big moustache and a tall flak-jacket that tickled his chin. He would ride the lead vehicle, a big white four-wheel-drive plastered with EU stickers. There were four more brand-new ECHO trucks and a half-dozen GMCs; powerful eight-seater tourers with tinted windows and deep upholstery, accessorised with TVs and CD players and air-conditioning, capable of high-speed driving on the desert highway.

The vehicles jockeyed through the city-centre traffic and picked up speed as we left town. I fell asleep, opening my eyes at dawn to see pale sand under a crust of rock like broken chocolate. Despite our early getaway the border was already a vast caravanserai of vehicles – GMCs with 'TV' lettered on the sides in fluorescent tape, beat-up taxis, trailer trucks and flash four-by-fours – besieging the buildings of the customs post. Aid workers and journalists stood around under the tin roof that shaded the inspection lanes. They wore identical outfits: hiking boots, combat trousers and many-pocketed waistcoats sporting the logos of news networks or humanitarian bodies. I chatted to a large American from an outfit called the Texas Food Bank, formed by some of that state's 'concerned restaurateurs' who'd donated their product to help the Iraqi people. This had been collected, flown at considerable expense to Amman and was now travelling in specially hired refrigerated trucks to Baghdad for distribution.

'Kinda like a thank-you from the US of A,' the man explained, 'for lettin' us bring them their freedom.'

An ill-tempered traffic jam marked the Iraqi side of the frontier, bunched on a gap in the concrete barrier where a solitary Iraqi guard screamed and gesticulated with his unloaded AK-47 at the jockeying trucks, sometimes pointing it at their contemptuous drivers. American soldiers – the first we'd seen – looked on from a raised plinth that bore a tiled portrait of Saddam Hussein, his eyes and moustache still quite perky under the fine film of mud that had been painted over his face. Bored travellers took out cameras to record the scene and the troops yelled in unison, 'No pictures!' with a harmony that suggested much recent practice. After a zigzag approach between stone barriers we stopped at the checkpoint, overseen by the heavy machine guns of a pair of parked Humvees. A soldier scanned our passports. 'One Jordanian', he called to a colleague in the sentry booth, 'One French. A Canadian. And ...' – he inspected the cover of my passport, front and back – 'a, uh, South Australian'.

Out of the border post, past a bronze statue of Saddam on horseback flanked by side-mounted missiles – an explosive charge had cut off the front legs, so that horse and rider were nose-dived like a fall at a steeplechase – we reached a pirate gasoline station of tanker-trucks parked on the sand, transferring fuel with hand pumps and taking payment in dollars. The fuel, tapped from some pipeline, was unrefined but our truck seemed to like it well enough, and soon our convoy was roaring along the six-lane desert highway at over a hundred miles an hour, the vehicles looping and hustling for position on the deserted blacktop. Buff-coloured plains spread out on either side. After an hour we crossed a concrete overpass, narrowed to a single lane by missile strikes that had turned much of the roadway into a sagging trampoline of reinforcing bar. A large touring bus sat in the tangle, its glass and metal rent by fragment-strikes. The road cut straight ahead through empty desert, the only milestones the occasional skeleton of another burned-out bus in a pool of seared tarmac. Where the highway skirted towns and intersections more were to be seen, their panels riddled, a brown stain percolated into the ground. Iraq's national bus service had made juicy targets on the smart-bomb guidance screens of Coalition aircraft fifteen thousand feet above, giving the passengers no chance of escape; they had, in military parlance, 'died in place'.

Despite the warnings about Ar-Ramadi, the moustached Belgian timed his petrol stop so that the ECHO vehicles had to refill just as we reached it. We halted by the roadside in a highly vulnerable configuration while jerrycans were emptied slowly through funnels and the ECHO security man looked nervously – with the rest of us – at the outskirts of the town and a nearby grove of date palms in which lurked some abandoned Iraqi armour. Black Hawk helicopters blattered overhead, patrolling the green swamp that lined the Euphrates. It was from this point that our Jordanian driver began to fret. Tripling his cigarette rate, he hunched down in his seat until, by the time we passed Falluja, he was peering beneath the steering wheel's arc. On the freeways that entered Baghdad, Iraqi tanks and personnel carriers stood at angles on the shoulder, their hatches open. I lifted my camera.

'No picture!' the driver screamed. 'Baghdad dangerous, see camera, shoot! Baghdad too dangerous!'

We appeared at greater risk from the convoys of US army trucks barrelling towards us on both sides of the road, headlights blazing and men in the top turrets clutching fifty-calibre machine guns with one hand and their carbines with the other as though uncertain which to fire first. Donkey carts and pickups piled with loot – armchairs, refrigerators, pyramids of doors – careered across our path through a brown fog, compounded of dust and the pall from burning oil-ditches that had been ignited during the war to create smoke-screens against enemy bombers and still smouldered somewhere to the south. We entered the city in a rush of vehicles and were swept up in a delirious switchback: hopping kerbs, cutting through converging traffic and backtracking up the wrong side of motorway ramps part-blocked by blasted armoured cars. Each traffic circle featured a Saddam statue, some pristine, others blown into a cubist scaffolding of the human form. Parks contained military trucks, tossed on end among the shredded trees. Taller buildings were burned-out shells or lay collapsed around stark columns. From the elevation of a bridge I saw the Information and Telecommunications Ministries, familiar from the TV war, holed by missile strikes. Beside the Tigris our road was narrowed by concrete blocks that forced us to a crawl. An Abrams tank covered our approach; others blocked side-streets behind glinting concertina wire. A mad-eyed boy in a US helmet and flak-jacket leaned into the car.

'Careful, man,' he said, jaw muscle throbbing, face black with grime and cammo paint, 'things just got stupid again.'

'Watch yourselves ahead,' elaborated his officer from a chair set up in the lee of the tank's hull, 'there's bang-bang down the road.'

Detouring through a deserted residential quarter, bumping over toppled barricades, we reached the compound of our hotel. The concrete tower-block was plastered ochre from the sandstorms that had left dunes in the bottom of the dry swimming pool. Tape criss-crossed the grimy windows, corridors and halls black after the outside glare. There was no electricity. We dropped our bags and shook hands with the two doctors from our group already there – a compact Frenchman and a doughy Serb – and then, tired, dehydrated and hungry, I was whisked by them directly to another of Baghdad's concrete towers for a meeting of the NGO Co-ordinating Committee for Iraq (NCCI). In the long room the sounds of traffic echoed like surf in a cave, so that the agency representatives, sitting along an endless table, could hear hardly a word each other said. The discussion was about a meeting between the committee and the US military. Co-ordination was in abeyance. There was, rather, a free fight: high principle – 'no one sits at my table with a gun' – versus moral righteousness: 'Our mission is to help. I will sit down with anyone who makes that possible'.

In the late afternoon heat, the windows admitting exhaust-haze and the crackle of shots, the same murk of rhetoric that had surrounded the military offensive seemed to be clouding the humanitarian response. Apart from some honourable exceptions, most of the organisations present had compromised their operational autonomy a year before, in their eagerness to get into Afghanistan, when Western governments had used humanitarian intervention – against the repressions of the fundamentalist Taleban, America's erstwhile ally – as a justification for war. These international aid groups had formed the humanitarian arm of the assault; 'a force multiplier for us', US Secretary of State Colin Powell had described them, 'such an important part of our combat team'. Now the same agencies were protesting about principle in a new war that – discounting the myths about Iraqi–Al-Qaeda collaboration and weapons of mass destruction – again justified itself as a military intervention on human rights grounds. Beside me a tall Frenchman watched the clamour over the tip of his cigarette.

'If you make yourself a prostitute', he observed dryly, 'you cannot reclaim your honour by arguing about the price'.

Back at our hotel some of the aid workers repaired to our room to continue the discussion. I'd hardly had a chance to talk to my new colleagues, but now, light-headed with fatigue, I studied them from my seat on the carpet. The small, dark-haired French doctor was an ex-fighter pilot – and seventh-best pistol shot in the world, he informed me   whose voice never lost its calm tenor, even under intense provocation. Some of this came from the Serb, whose expressive range stretched from deepest melodrama – 'I ham here for people of Iraq' – to heart-stopping hyperbole: 'Tomorrow you are goink into area of city vere vill try to shoot you. Is more dangerous zan playink Russian Roulette with *five* (hand raised, chubby fingers spread), yes, *five* bullets'.

If I was to deal with danger the next morning I would need to sleep, but the meeting showed no signs of abating. I excused myself and took the stairs to the hotel roof. The air was hot and close and lacked all power to refresh.

I would soon become familiar with that breathless night and the view over the blacked-out city. The darkness was accentuated by the muted glow of paraffin lamps in nearby windows, and the odd building with its own generator flooded in light. Beyond lay voids of emptiness where the war was being played out: a blast across the river, orange flames to the south-east. Lightless helicopters passed overhead and red tracer rose near the university. Journalists, aid workers and mysterious contactors walked complex paths across the rooftop asphalt as they spoke into sat-phones whose reception flared and faded. Along the parapet the correspondents hunched in the glow of their laptops, filing copy or receiving editorial instruction through satellite email links. I tried to call my landlady and on the third try got through. I explained that I was now in Baghdad, unable to move my stuff out of her flat until I got back.

'What's that noise?'

'Shooting,' I explained.

'Why is there shooting?' she demanded. Again I mentioned the war and my work, and asked that she consider an extension so that I could find new accommodation when I returned.

'We'll see,' she replied, and the connection was cut.

Sometime in the depths of the night I was roused by what sounded like cannon-fire, each report ringing through the walls, and again at the time of the dawn prayers when the mullah's incantations were overlaid by the discord of a machine gun firing in short bursts.

After joining my colleagues at the hotel's repast of thin coffee and hard bread, we set off with our driver to the Ministry of Health. It lay in the northern part of the city near the river. The iron gates had been flattened by a tank, but its façade still carried a great billboard of Saddam patting the head of a bed-bound patient. The building itself was a looted, twelve-floor shell, its interior partitions stitched with bullet holes. Every document in the place had been dumped from the windows. They formed a hill of papers that lapped up to the sills and extended in drifts through the grounds; tables of malaria rates and nutritional data jumbled with employment records, indents for thermometers and the colour prints from pathology books. Staff members had found a blackboard ripped from a lecture-hall and were using it as a skip to haul away rubble. Others wandered through the mounds of paper, picking up a graph here, an X-ray plate elsewhere and staring at the items as though trying to imagine how they could ever again fit together.

My French colleague introduced me to Dr Sadek of the Department of Preventive Medicine. As we talked, US military police armoured vehicles rolled through the gates. The Iraqi doctor's face twitched. Dismounting, the MPs formed a cordon around the vehicles while their passengers – a contingent of army medical officers – buckled on helmets and pistols and marched into the building's dark interior. The MP escort was taking no chances; a convoy of military doctors had been ambushed nearby the day before, with eleven wounded. A Heath Ministry director entering the gates was pulled from his car. When a search revealed a pistol under the seat – 'Everyone needs protection in these times,' Dr Sadek growled – the man was thrown to the ground and handcuffed before being hustled away. The parking lot contained some ministry vehicles saved from or not yet hijacked by the looters: trucks, ambulances, a few official cars. The soldiers started deposing the Health Ministry transport from its place, ordering drivers to move the vehicles out into the dangerous streets. From above descended a rain of ash, carried by the wind that gusted through burned-out buildings.

✪

Pending surgical employment, I found myself working with my medical group at the opposite end of the clinical spectrum: primary health care, basic intervention to try to prevent disease rather than the resource-intensive surgical treatment of injuries in which I was experienced. In the 1960s Iraq's ruling socialist Ba'ath Party had set up a network of around thirteen hundred primary health-care clinics in cities, towns and villages across the country as part of a programme – including schooling and medical care – for the secularisation of Iraqi society; particularly the Shi'a majority, who were generally poorer, less educated and more strongly under the sway of their mullahs. Until the 1991 Gulf War these clinics had provided a free GP service, treating coughs and colds, immunising babies and carrying out ante-natal assessments. As Iraq became increasingly impoverished with the imposition of sanctions, the clinics had run satellite care centres in schools, where nutritionists distributed UN-provided food supplements and sent significantly malnourished children to therapeutic feeding centres in the hospitals. With the health service too starved of resources, patients became required to pay a small fee, which was remitted by each clinic to the government pharmaceutical supplier in return for its monthly drug consignment. A degree of corruption entered the system, but for the poorer half of Baghdad's six million people, for perhaps around two-thirds of Iraqis across the country, the clinics remained the only health care there was.

Throughout the war they had kept running, tending wounds and infections. Drugs and dressings, basic at the best of times, ran low in the treatment of casualties. Clinics had been looted in the rioting that followed the American arrival, some wrecked. Despite the

Occupation Force patrols on Baghdad's main thoroughfares, their survival remained precarious, but it was difficult to know the extent of the problem; there were no telephones, no fuel supplies for official transport, and Health Ministry vehicles were being snatched by armed gangs. The Departments of Primary Health Care and Preventive Medicine had been the first in the Health Ministry to reopen, sweeping debris from their eleventh-floor offices and compiling lists from memory to replace those lost when computers and files had vanished along with chairs and desks. My two colleagues had made contact with them to arrange a plan for finding out how much of the primary health-care clinic network still functioned. Now we headed upstairs for a group meeting. The Frenchman sped like a terrier up the narrow concrete staircase, cleaving through the throng that froze to the wall where the handrail was missing or bunched behind puffing bureaucrats. Four floors below us the Serb stumped upwards, radiating resentment at the enforced exercise.

Our Iraqi counterparts were young and middle-aged, women and men, in every way like doctors I'd worked with around the world. Several, like Dr Sadek, had overseas qualifications. They all spoke English and greeted us with great courtesy. Our first project required teams, consisting of one member of our group and two Ministry of Health doctors, to carry out a detailed assessment of each of the 167 clinics in Baghdad and identify crucial shortfalls – structural, material and personnel – that we would try to help through our emergency aid programme. I was also required to visit hospitals in order to identify which ones could accept patients, including surgical trauma, referred from the clinics. It was clear that these tasks, though for me not as personally fulfilling as surgery, were probably more constructive in the chaotic conditions of occupied Baghdad. I was partnered with two women doctors – calm Dr Saria and small, expressive Dr Hanna – and we set off with our list of assigned clinics in a Ministry of Health truck.

I sat beside the driver as he braved the currents of traffic, skirting angry whirlpools where US tanks had blocked an intersection and avoiding the long doldrums of the queues for gas. From the back seat my new colleagues questioned me on my origins, prospects and what languages I spoke, and tut-tutted at my remissness in failing to get married. The doctors were beneficiaries of Ba'athist policy on the education of women that had given Iraq the highest percentage of female doctors and scientists in the Middle East. Both were pleased that Saddam was gone, but concerned about the future of the secular society in which they'd hoped their children would grow up. The truck traversed street after street of rough, low-roofed buildings with the occasional jutting finger of a mosque. Off the main through-routes the roads were dust, turned to swamp in places by the effluvium from sewage pipes fractured by the bombing. Children played amidst smouldering garbage and gutted army trucks. The two million Shi'a Muslims living in this quarter of east Baghdad had originally named it Sadr City after their revered religious leader, Mohammad Al-Sadr. Following the 1958 army rebellion that deposed the Iraqi monarchy and nationalised the oil fields, it became Al-Thawra – Revolution – City. A CIA-facilitated coup then brought the Ba'athists to power, but to the dismay of their US backers they'd failed to reverse the oil nationalisation and instead brought in a programme of socialist reforms. Revolution City kept its name until Saddam Hussein seized control of the Party in 1979, when the endless slums were named Saddam City. Now it had begun reverting to old appellations. The doctors called it Al-Thawra; Sadr City, insisted the local Shi'a religious movements regrouping around Al-Sadr's firebrand nephew Moqtada.

At the first neighbourhood clinic the medical director was justifiably proud; she'd managed to keep the place operating throughout the air-strikes, when its courtyard had been turned into a ward for the care of bombing victims. During the looting that followed, the clinic had had its doors smashed, its contents ransacked; the director could only berate the thieves as they made off with examination couches, microscopes and dental instruments. But somehow the clinic continued to function, tending sick infants, dressing bullet wounds and treating the first of the season's cases of typhoid. Now she was trying to prepare for anticipated cholera outbreaks while looking after her six-year-old son, whom she'd bring to work each day until the schools were running. The immunisation clinic was full of black-swathed women clutching babies that lacked any plumpness and watched us over their mothers' shoulders, heads nodding on scrawny necks. There were no vaccines, so the nurse was simply noting names until the day when supplies returned. My Ministry of Health colleagues went off to make an inventory of the few supplies in the pharmacy, while I accompanied the director to obtain a bacteriological sample from the standpipe at the compound gate that provided the clinic with an intermittent trickle of water.

From the street there came a tearing burst of gunfire. While I was still registering the noise she was already dashing for cover, hand on her boy's head to keep him low. I glimpsed their faces – hers tight with tension, his turned back to look at her in fear – as they ran. Beside me the clinic guard had flattened himself against the gatepost, his weapon raised; now he called up to some men on the roof of the building opposite, their own guns ready, who peered along the street. There were scattered shots, then silence. The director returned, a tremulous smile on her face.

'Sorry, Doctor.' She pressed a hand to her chest and laughed nervously. 'Too much shooting.'

Back in her office she kept the child tightly clasped as she continued to tell me about her fears of a pending epidemic: ruptured water and sewage mains mingling their contents underground and people crowding into the surrounding tenements from bombed areas to the east.

In the old days, she explained, there had been a protocol if they detected communicable diseases; the Ministry of Health would be informed, samples sent to the Central Public Health Laboratory and epidemiologists mobilised. Now there were no sample-tubes to send specimens, no means of transporting them, no telephone links to notify of an outbreak and drugs to combat contagious illness were in short supply.

'We cannot even offer tea,' she said. 'The looters took the kettle and the cups.'

Isolated in Al-Thawra, she could not know quite how devastated were the institutions on which she had previously depended. The Public Health Laboratory had been torched, its centrifuges and microscopes fused by the heat. Only the government drug warehouses were still substantially intact, their contents protected from rampaging gangs by their guards, but the old bureaucracy had also survived; without the right requisition form and payment, no stocks were being released.

☉

The health system was just a small part of the ruin. Apart from the Oil Ministry, protected by American troops, all other government institutions – Finance, Education, Telecommunications; museums, power stations, sewage works and water plants – had been left to looters, who were stripping out every vestige of usable material and burning the rest. Iraq had been studied exhaustively by Pentagon planners from before the first Gulf War and its subjugation had been the primary goal of Republican foreign policy-planning documents since 1997. It seemed inconceivable that no strategy existed to restore order in Baghdad. Aid workers and journalists, even some of my Iraqi medical colleagues, suggested that the chaos was a sophisticated programme of destabilisation designed to shake up Iraqi society and encourage factions to promote their own agendas and leaders; as these emerged they could either be co-opted by the Coalition Provisional Authority (CPA) or destroyed. Yet the void continued, with different groups vying for control of medical facilities: Shi'a Islamic bodies, the KDP and PUK Kurdish factions whose forces had come into the capital from the north on the heels of retreating Iraqi units, and the Iraqi National Congress of exile Ahmed Chalabi, who now arrived in Baghdad promising that his White House backers would guarantee medical services and doctors' salaries. A hospital director that I'd met in the morning might have been deposed by the candidate of a rival movement when I returned at noon – sometimes two or three pretenders would be holding court simultaneously in different offices – while the injured bled on the floor and desperate mothers roamed the corridors, collapsed babies in their arms, crying for medicine.

The Shi'a organisations, expecting that the American-appointed Iraqi Governing Council would leave them marginalized, were already taking over services in the parts of the city where they predominated. They had bitter experience of the US. In 1991, following the retreat of Saddam's army in the face of the Allied ground assault, the Shi'a had risen up in their holy cities in southern Iraq and danced in the streets. America had been fearful of an Iranian-style Islamic revolution and elected to allow the Republican Guard free rein in putting down the insurgency. The mass-graves of that atrocity were now being opened, yielding up the first of an estimated three hundred thousand bodies. In Baghdad's Shi'a neighbourhoods their affiliation would be flagged by an electricity pylon or the plinth for a Saddam statue carrying the black and green banners of Shi'a movements – Al-Hawsa or Al-Dawa or the Mahdi Army of Al-Sadr – and portraits of their clerics, guarded by local militia. Men with beards and AK-47s controlled the gates to the clinics and my arrival was greeted sometimes with anger or the thrust of a gun-barrel against my chest.

'*Amrikya*'! they shouted, '*Britaniya*'!

I would explain that I was from South Africa. '*Jinub Afriqye*', I would say. 'Nelson Mandela'. His public opposition to the war was known throughout Iraq, and the hard faces would relax. The local mullah – tall and grave, turbaned and robed in black or rust – would want to know the reason for our visit. I'd explain that I was a volunteer doctor from overseas, working with Ministry of Health personnel to conduct an assessment of clinic needs. Mention of the Ministry of Health or foreign aid would evoke suspicion, sometimes rage.

'They must stay away from here! We are providing for our people,' the mullah might shout, and we'd be hustled off to be shown the pharmacy, stocked with cartons of drugs donated by the mosque, dispensed from a table lent by the mosque.

Medical colleagues at the NGO Co-ordinating Committee meetings reported similar encounters with increasingly militant Shi'a groups. Women health workers in primary health-care centres were being forced to wear headscarves and some complained that clerics were against women working at all. In one clinic the female doctors who'd run it had been evicted, with medical care now being provided by an appropriately devout junior medical student. The failure of the CPA to restore basic services was strengthening the power of Shi'a bodies that provided social support – health care, shelter, aid to the poor – in place of the state institutions that previously saw to these requirements. A French doctor who had worked in Beirut reminded us how the Shi'a group Hizbollah, that called itself the Organisation of the Oppressed on Earth, had been unknown in the Lebanon until the 1982 Israeli invasion. During the void in civic order under Israeli occupation, Hizbollah collected taxes, supplied social services and medical care. Its resultant popularity and political strength built the organisation into a powerful military force that eventually drove Israel from southern Lebanon.

✛

Driving through the city in the early morning, smoke hanging like a wall at the end of streets, banks of stink from rotting garbage and fractured sewers and black shit-lakes overlapping the curbs, I was trying to get to a municipality to the south of the city. The river bridges had been blown up by Iraqi forces to slow the American advance and in a couple of places US Army engineers had thrown up a Bailey Bridge or floating roadway, where we joined the long queues of local transport trying to cross. Sometimes our driver left the highway to seek back-routes through fields and villages, passing bombed bunkers and undamaged Iraqi missiles on launch trailers under the trees. Marines held this sector and were being shot at every night. Their vehicles were parked in rows among the date palms, with sandbagged gun-pits at the borders of their encampment. In the town they had placed tanks across the streets to force the packed, heat-flayed traffic of sagging pickup trucks and overloaded donkey-carts into single file. This was where US forces had faced the greatest resistance when entering Baghdad – it was said that six thousand Iraqi troops had died here in the defence of the city – and walls bore the star-shaped scars of rocket-propelled grenades.

The district hospital had been bomb-damaged, looted and subsequently returned to some degree of function by the Madrassah religious school of a nearby mosque. A day before there had been a huge explosion in a US Army–guarded ordnance dump in the neighbourhood. The Americans blamed it on an attack by Saddam loyalists and the community blamed US forces for storing bombs and missiles in a residential area, but whatever the issues, the blast had killed a number of civilians and injured many more who now lay on the hospital's wards. Emotions were high, the place full of angry young zealots with shaven heads. We passed with difficulty through a chanting, fist-waving group at the door – the Iraqi woman doctor I was with hastily donned a headscarf – and made our way to the medical director's office. He explained the demonstrators' demands: America had injured their people, the mosque had saved them by providing hospital resources where the Ministry of Health had failed, and now they wanted to run the hospital and dictate who should work there. As we spoke, the noise increased to a crescendo of shouting; along the corridor a struggle was in progress. A man escaped from the blows and dashed into the office, shirt torn and his face bruised.

The doors had been blown from their hinges or smashed down by looters and there was no way to bar the mob who pushed into the office and pressed at the windows with their chanted denunciations. The director placed himself in front of his beaten colleague, speaking persuasively. Eventually the men withdrew, muttering, while the doctor who had been assaulted trembled and fumed at these 'backward thinkers' who were dictating how he should do his work. A short while later at the doorway to the wards I was forcibly prevented – with a blow to the chest and more shouting – from entering; as well as the fact that I was an unbeliever, there was an objection to male doctors attending female patients. Further persuasion from the director was needed before I was allowed to pass through into wards full of hollow-cheeked babies dehydrated from gastro-enteritis, and victims of the ordnance explosion.

I found the Iraqi surgeon busy assessing one of them, a twelve-year-old boy with his face and body flayed by multiple puncture wounds. These appeared to be from bits of the environment – brick-chips, pebbles, flakes of charcoal – that had been blown through the skin, beneath which they lay like gritty tattoos. Fortunately he had turned his head away at the instant of explosion so that he was not blinded, and his eyes flicked fearfully between our faces as we discussed, in English, his clinical condition. The child's fever might have been due to infection from dirt that the projectiles had carried in, and the pain of the punctures could explain why his stomach muscles were tense, but the surgeon was concerned that there might be perforations through the abdominal wall into the gut. It was essential that possible peritonitis not be overlooked, and without electricity we lacked even the limited diagnostic assistance of an X-ray, so we took him to the operating room to explore his lacerations. An anaesthetic nurse administered sedation, light enough that the boy flinched and whimpered in his sleep as we cleaned his wounds with scrubbing-brushes. The larger ones we probed to see how deep they were, washing out the debris with clean water that had been supplied, in plastic bags, for drinking purposes by the Red Cross.

There is a procedure called diagnostic peritoneal lavage which is used to detect leakage from the gut or bleeding into the belly. It involves the insertion of a cannula into the abdominal cavity just below the umbilicus. The test is not prescribed for children – because the thinner-walled intestine, lying closely together, is at risk of damage from the cannula needle – but we were trying to avoid laparotomy (open surgery) unless it was absolutely necessary and so the risk seemed worth taking. I passed a catheter to empty the bladder so that it would be out of the way of the needle, which I stuck carefully through the thin muscle of the abdomen. Half a litre of saline, suspended from a drip stand, was gently infused. Then I laid the saline container on the floor so that the fluid could flow back into the transparent bag. A significant finding would be the presence of shreds of bowel content or of blood, indicated by a shade of redness traditionally described as 'darker than a page of the *Financial Times*'; in his training the Iraqi surgeon heard of this definition, but had never seen the actual newspaper. We watched the saline titrate slowly out of the belly and into the bag. From the courtyard came a sound of wood splintering, as an orderly kicked to pieces an ammunition box in case a fire was needed to sterilise the instruments. Gunfire swung around the horizon like a compass-hand.

☉

Only a few children's hospitals and specialist centres had acquired US military protection and these were the favoured recipients of attention from the aid organisations. On the occasions that I had to visit these places I would find representatives from two or three medical relief groups waiting to be received by the hospital directors, who would endure politely meeting after meeting, their entire day taken up with requests for data, statistics and bed-numbers – for those vital field-reports – or finding storage space for the imminent delivery of charity truckloads of therapeutic material. TV crews would be in place to film the boxes being passed hand-to-hand into the building, the logo of the aid organisation catching the light. Sometimes the contents turned out to be junk, having been donated by overseas drug companies and medical equipment manufacturers only too pleased finally to clear those low-demand, date-expired products out of their warehouses and claim the tax write-off at the same time.

But the CPA did have plans for Iraq's health system, as I discovered when I attended a meeting on the issue in the Ministry of Health. The main auditorium had been cleaned out, chairs found, a generator set up to supply power for the microphone and the directorships invited of each of the ministry's departments. Armed US soldiers stood against the walls under poster-sized copies of a proclamation from the Commander, Coalition Ground Forces in Iraq. 'I charge the citizens of Iraq to immediately return to work', it read. 'Citizens who have served in leadership roles must identify themselves to Coalition Forces to assist in the building of a new Iraqi government'. A preppy type in button-down shirt and chinos, from the CPA's 'reconstruction' subsidiary – the Office for Rehabilitation and Humanitarian Assistance (ORHA) – stood at the podium. The projection screen behind him, torn into expressionist shapes where looters had thrown the furniture through it, gave the scene a rather surreal air.

'My first objective is to facilitate a transparent democratic process,' said the ORHA official. He introduced the man he'd just nominated as interim Minister of Health. 'I will appoint all new directors-general and directors in the Ministry of Health, based on the recommendations of the interim minister.'

Awed by the transparency of this democracy, the audience murmured; the interim minister was an unliked ex-brigadier in the Iraqi army medical service who had prospered under Saddam's regime. Forms were then distributed, to be completed by all department directors and countersigned by two witnesses. Headed 'Final Victory' and written in English and Arabic, they came in two versions: a declaration – 'I am not, nor have I ever been, a member of the Ba'ath Party' – or a renunciation – 'I hereby disavow and renounce my membership in the Ba'ath Party'. Each director was also required to write out a biography listing previous posts and responsibilities. Voices were raised in consternation as people realised that their careers and futures could depend on these bits of paper. Many had joined the party in the 1960s and '70s in support of its social programmes, long before Saddam had warped its purpose to his own ends. The man from ORHA seemed surprised at this hiccup in the progress of his forum and, somewhat irritated, he conferred with the military. A colonel of the US Army Medical Corps mounted the podium, pistol on his thigh, and demanded the forms – 'for administrative purposes' – be completed and returned in ten minutes.

Then a core aspect of health reform was addressed: the opening of medical provision to market forces. A new pay scale for government hospital doctors would reward specialisation with the freedom to expand their private practice. Conditions for those working in preventive medicine, public health and primary health care would also change. Instead of the solid Ministry of Health salaries they'd received in the past, designed to encourage a lifetime career in public service, they too would be offered the 'flexibility' of diversifying into private practice.

'Revolutionary changes for health care in Iraq,' declared the ORHA convenor.

From the audience, doctors interjected. They'd not been paid in the last ten weeks, during which they'd treated thousands of wounded and stayed on duty twenty-four hours a day guarding medical facilities. Damage from looting could not be repaired, insecurity was growing, water supplies contaminated, communicable disease on the rise and the vaccination programme had collapsed, while essential supplies were not being released by the government drug warehouses. Facilities were increasingly falling outside the control of the Ministry of Health or being replaced by clinics in nearby mosques. What, they demanded, was being done to address these immediate issues?

'Everything will go back to the old system,' said the interim minister firmly. 'End of matter.'

The ex-brigadier's grasp of developments was no more secure than that on his job: within thirty-six hours he was forced to stand down when Ministry of Health staff demonstrated against his closeness to Saddam Hussein. A few days later ORHA ceased to exist, its functions subsumed into the CPA, and its head, General Jay Garner, recalled home. His replacement, Proconsul Paul Bremer, wore suits with aviator shades and desert boots and carried orders from Washington to stamp down firmly. The forms regarding Ba'ath Party membership were his first reading matter. Bremer's Order Number One, the de-Ba'athification decree, expelled fifty thousand ex-members of the party from government service. The expertise of senior administrators, Health Ministry officials, professors of medicals schools, hospital directors and heads of universities was discarded. Simultaneously Bremer disbanded the four-hundred-thousand-strong Iraqi army, filling the streets with angry ex-soldiers who had no skills to fall back on but their weapons training.

☉

The official account of what was happening in Iraq could be heard at the daily CMCC (Civil/Military Co-ordination Committee) meeting, held at five P.M. within the fortified precincts of Coalition Headquarters in the Republican Palace. Someone from our group was detailed to attend these meetings – known, inevitably, as the 'five o'clock follies' after the richly derided US military briefings in Saigon during the Vietnam War – and when not occupied in clinics or hospitals, I sometimes went along. The palace complex, Saddam's old presidential headquarters, occupied a five-square-mile elbow of the Tigris' west bank. From its sandbagged gates, and over the Tamuz Bridge to the south that was blocked to all but US military traffic, now issued the armoured patrols of Baghdad's liberators. We'd approach the palace over the Jumhuriya Bridge, the lowering sun dim through the smoke of buildings burning in the western suburbs, and swing into the northern entrance to be searched. Leaving our vehicle, doors open, trunk and bonnet raised, to be poked through by soldiers, we were patted down beneath the lowered muzzle of an Abrams tank. A grand triumphal archway – covered a hundred yards back by another tank – was the entrance to the palace grounds, a quarter of gardens, council chambers, reception halls and residences now occupied by the country's new rulers.

The meetings were held in a carved-wood and marble hall previously used by Saddam for receiving dignitaries. The toilets could not be flushed because there was no water, but it was opulently furnished with gold and white Louise Quatorze armchairs whose volutes snagged the holsters of the American officers. The leaders of the aid groups sat at a long banqueting table, their rank and file sharing the walls with note-taking army lieutenants, while the colonels gave us Good News. The CPA was launching a new TV station, broadcast in Arabic with American music and advertising, a 'lifestyle' channel intended to counter 'the negative images and journalistic self-censorship' of Al-Jazeera Arabic Television (subsequently banned by the US-appointed Iraq Governing Counsel). Another American corporation would be setting up a cell-phone service to replace the bombed national telecommunications network, which was not planned for restoration. Electricity supply, sanitation and water quality would soon reach standards higher than ever attained under the previous regime, though this colonel professed a problem: armed looters continued to target the plants, and the US-appointed civilian guards, despite their dollar-a-day stipend, tended to run away.

'So would I,' said one of the aid workers. 'Civilians aren't going to die to protect those facilities.'

'But how did they protect the facilities before?' asked the officer, perplexed.

'There wasn't a problem before. The country had a government.'

Another intriguing part of the CMCC meetings was the daily security briefing, which we hoped might give us some advance knowledge of the danger levels in the parts of the city where we operated. A map of Baghdad would be projected on the wall, divided into colour-coded sectors. Green, or 'permissive', ones had reported no 'contacts with enemy forces' in the previous twenty-four hours;

yellow – 'uncertain' – areas had seen one or two incidents; and in the red, or 'hostile', zones there had been three attacks or more. It would be announced that security was improving, with Baghdad currently showing no 'hostile' areas, though a glance at the map would reveal that 'uncertain' ones had increased from seven to fifteen overnight.

'Paramilitary resistance continues to decrease across the country,' the officer would beam, then gabble through a list of incidents – a US vehicle blown up on the airport road, five hundred mines found in Abu Wahid, a patrol shot at in Abu Qadair, a soldier hit by a sniper in Al-Karadah, two humanitarian organisation vehicles hijacked and an rocket-propelled grenade fired at American troops in Al-Jihad – quite at odds with the smile that did not leave his face.

There was never any mention of Iraqi dead, though the clinics constantly received civilian casualties. I'd arrived at a clinic to find the staff clustered around two small girls pale with terror and blood-loss; the only survivors of a family whose car had been riddled with gunfire. In the courtyard women shrieked and clawed at their faces in grief. We set up IV drips on the children while a vehicle was found to take them to a hospital. Then, at the clinic director's request, I'd gone to talk to the troops manning the local checkpoint where the incident had occurred. The road was deserted apart from a small white car on deflated tyres, its windows shot out. At the corner, behind a barrier of concertina wire, stood some Armoured Fighting Vehicles. I walked slowly forward, my hands in clear view, holding high the ID letter from my medical organisation. The American soldiers watched my approach through their wrap-round sunglasses.

'I'm a doctor with an international aid group,' I explained to a sergeant. 'May I speak to your officer?'

A cheery-looking young lieutenant appeared and stuck out his hand. 'Hey, Doc. What can we do for you?'

I stayed on the outside of the wire.

'Look, please understand if I don't shake hands,' I said. 'Everyone around here is upset about the people who were shot.' I pointed at the white car. 'I'm working at the clinic up the road, and it's better if the neighbourhood sees me as being sort of neutral with you guys.'

'Yeah. Sure.' The officer put his hand behind his back. I could see that he was offended.

'It's they own fault,' said the sergeant. 'They shoulda stop a hundred metres away, like it says in the rules of engagement.'

'They're civilians,' I objected, 'they don't understand about rules of engagement.'

A soldier looked down at me from the nearest Bradley. There was a bulge of chewing tobacco in his lower lip.

'Civilians my ass,' he growled. 'These fuckin' ragheads did Nine-Eleven.'

✚

Yet another version of reality could be gleaned from the journalists whom I spoke to back at the hotel in the evenings, after they'd been out all day pursuing the real issues identified by their head-office editors. One day the lead would be the mass graves, and reporters slouched in from having spent the day at exhumations, dirty and drained and trumping each others' accounts of how many corpses they'd seen. Forty-eight hours later the dead were *passé* and the breaking story was the rehabilitation of the Iraqi police force, which had the news crews elbowing each other to interview the four cops on traffic duty near the central railway station: the only visible evidence of the CPA's claims that ten thousand or fifteen thousand or twenty-three thousand policemen were back at their posts. Another epic news-event was the arrival of a cavalcade of armoured Humvees at the Ministry of Sport and Recreation – partly burned, thoroughly looted – where a colonel and two majors had dismounted behind a screen of military police to announce to the media the revitalisation of the Iraqi Olympic Committee with a grant to purchase track suits for the restoration of national sporting pride. There was a recurring vogue for up-beat stories about Ahmed Chalabi as Iraq's future leader.

Chalabi hadn't been in Baghdad since the fifties and was widely mistrusted by the CIA and the State Department, who accused him of purloining US government funds meant for the Iraqi resistance, while a Jordanian court had sentenced him to prison for the embezzlement of over fifty million dollars. But the Pentagon still saw his exile INC (Iraqi National Congress) as the country's government-in-waiting and Chalabi himself as its new president, who would make peace with Israel, and war – if so directed – with Iran. The Free Iraqi Forces, Chalabi's seven-hundred-strong US-equipped militia, was supposed to form the core of the new Iraqi army. The senior FIF officers were quartered in our hotel, but after a few had been killed in an attack on their convoy, they only went out protected by US armour. There were reports of INC officials requisitioning prime properties – villas and business premises – in the city, as well as vehicles and matériel; one health centre director showed me his clinic's electrical generator that he had been ordered to give up to the head of security at the local INC headquarters.

'They have already taken the batteries so we cannot start it,' said the director. 'They say they will send a truck for the generator.' He looked sadly at the machine. 'We received this generator just before the war, under the UN oil-for-food programme, and we guarded it ourselves from the looters. Without it the clinic cannot run.'

I recounted the clinic director's story to a newly arrived correspondent, busy setting up his satellite email link, and suggested he interview the man.

'Sorry, can't use it,' he said. 'I'm here to cover the "reconstruction of Iraq" angle.'

Nobody seemed keen to address the big story in town, about who was responsible for the escalating attacks against US forces. A journalist described to me how he had been caught in traffic at an army checkpoint on the North Bridge when he'd seen a man step out of the throng on the pavement, put a pistol against the neck of a soldier and fire without breaking stride. The shooter vanished at once among the crowd while the other soldiers ducked and dashed around trying to work out where the shot had come from, and their squad-mate died at their feet. At an army press briefing later that day the journalist had tried to open a discussion about this and other incidents, but though he raised his hand and asked his question clearly and succinctly, it fell into a well of silence. The colonel stood on tip-toe, craning his neck to see the back of the hall.

'Yes?' he said. 'The lady from Fox?' and the tension was broken with a question about a football match played between the Marines and Iraqi schoolchildren.

RPG attacks spread like brushfire through the city, blasting open the lightly armoured Humvees. Huge Abrams tanks, previously parked in fixed positions, were more and more to be seen grinding along the streets. Red-cross-painted Casevac choppers clattered overhead. At the CMCC meetings the number of permissive, uncertain and hostile zones about the city fluctuated daily – sometimes a hitherto red zone would go orange, while three that were green yesterday switched to a warmer wavelength – but the trend was implacably upward. The CMCC fretted about how to deal with this problem and then decided that it was a presentational one. Red or hostile sectors were re-defined as those where there had been five or more 'contacts with enemy forces' in the previous twenty-four hours; two to four incidents now warranted merely an yellow 'uncertain' label, and any district where there had been no more than one fire-fight, RPG ambush or landmine could be happily described as permissive. At a stroke the map of Baghdad once again showed green amidst the hot zones. The descriptions of the incidents behind these figures acquired an ever more surreal quality – buildings 'went on fire'; shots were 'intercepted'; a patrol 'experienced an explosion situation' – as though the US forces were fighting ghosts.

While the situation on the streets became daily more precarious, the CPA was expanding and flourishing. The perimeter of the American Zone had enlarged far beyond the Republican Palace, to annex conference centres, hotels and stadiums. Civil/Military Affairs officers, intelligence operatives and technical specialists from the crack weapons-of-mass-destruction search teams had to be accommodated, along with consultants and contractors employed by the myriad US corporations working in Iraq. Generators chugged on the footpaths, trucks unloaded containers of computers, air-conditioners and toilet paper that were immediately absorbed inside the buildings. Palace halls were partitioned with board to make offices that duplicated and replaced the Iraqi government ministries: here was Finance; there, Power; along a corridor past the backed-up toilets,

Health. The Humvees lined along the boulevards of the palace grounds grew into double- and triple-parked queues, anointed with the divisional symbols of a score of units. On the kerbs, groups of lardy rear-echelon types and reservists jogged sluggishly in the afternoon heat.

At the same time, the number of humanitarian organisations attending the daily CMCC briefings was growing exponentially. Advocacy groups, human rights movements and development bodies that had been waiting on the sidelines in Amman and Kuwait City now flooded into Baghdad, extravagant with ideals and plans. Their delegates packed the hall and fought each other for CPA press releases, taking as many copies as they could grab. In the mêlée the last of Saddam's cut-glass-look gold-rimmed goblets smashed on the marble floor. These second-wave groups had lovely names: Peace Wings International, Earth Network, Compassion for Innocent Victims in Conflict, Life for Relief and Development, Human Relief Foundation, Solidarity for Peacemaking and Sharing, the International Consortium of Solidarity, Human Appeal International, Strategic World Impact, Global Care, Oasis of Love, Peace Volunteers and The Good People. It seemed churlish to begrudge them their debuts on the Baghdad stage, but some of them were frankly weird.

One of the evangelical groups wore bright yellow T-shirts showing a figure astride the globe with a Bible raised in one hand and a crucifix in the other, insensitive attire in any Muslim country and exquisitely provocative in Iraq. A Korean agency had a consignment of sixty tons of winter clothing that they wished to distribute even as spring temperatures reached the mid-forties centigrade; it would be ten degrees hotter by mid-summer. The Japanese seemed very young, with scant experience of humanitarian work – their country had perhaps the lowest rate in the world of giving sanctuary to refugees (fourteen souls admitted in the year 2000) – or the dangers of war; a baggage handler at Amman Airport had recently been killed by a mortar bomb in the suitcase of a Japanese journalist, who was taking it home as a souvenir.

At one meeting a couple of the new humanitarian groups had a request: they wanted the CPA to grant authorisation for them to carry guns in the course of their work. The American colonel seemed to favour the idea, asking all interested agencies to submit written notification so that the CPA could register them. Those of us who objected that there were already enough dangers in Baghdad without armed altruists, were told by the colonel that the US had no jurisdiction over the right of international aid organisations to bear weapons.

'But you're the government in Iraq right now,' we argued. 'You're the law here. You don't permit Iraqis to carry guns for their protection, so how can you let these people become a militia?'

At the next CMCC meeting we demanded to know which organisations had applied to be armed so that we could stay away from their operations and vehicles. The colonel disclosed that there'd been requests from three groups so far, though he refused to reveal their identities. He was then questioned about rumours that shots had been fired north of Baghdad from the vehicles of an aid convoy (one with 'peace' in its name) at some men beside the road ahead whom they'd suspected might be bandits. The colonel mumbled that he'd heard about it, and admitted that as a consequence the next aid vehicles using the road might be greeted with RPGs. Official sanction for the carrying of arms was quietly shelved.

✪

Perhaps, though, the distinction between humanitarian and military roles in Iraq was already terminally blurred. The UN, having been allowed by the Pentagon to reoccupy their old Baghdad headquarters at the Canal Hotel, were guarded by US Army Humvees whose machine guns were trained up and down the long avenue. Soldiers filled the tables in the hotel dining hall and lounged on sofas in the entrance lobby under bas-relief winged lions copied from the gates of Babylon. The main hall in which UN briefings were held was separated by glass doors from an area used for recreation by American troops. Inside it a translucent green roof admitted an underwater light that bathed the marble floor. Potted plants resembled aquarium décor. A TV set must have occupied the corner out of sight, for the soldiers all stood facing the same way, drifting a little in the manner of a school of basking sharks, the black butts of their shouldered weapons protruding like fins.

The UN security officers had served in Mozambique and Colombia, and their concerns reflected experience in countries suffering 'post-conflict instability' where the main threats were armed robbery and traffic accidents. They talked now of a worrying trend: Iraqis employed by the UN were receiving death threats from Islamic groups. 'By working with the unbelievers', read a message sent to a female clerk, 'you will be liable for powerful justice', ranging from 'the fate that cannot be named' to the killing of her family. Another had been ordered by the People's Punishment Committee to 'stop these things that are against Islam, or you will pay a very high price'. There followed a list of violent options. 'Remember', it ended unconvincingly, 'that the door of Allah's mercy is always open'.

But there were things happening in Iraq to infuriate even its most secular citizens. Daily, new contracts were being announced as every sector of the Iraqi economy was parcelled out to US companies. Halliburton, American Vice-President Cheney's ex-firm, got the largest tranche at $7 billion to run the oil fields for the next few years. Defence contractor Bechtel received $680 million for 'infrastructure projects'. Military contractor Dynacorp obtained a multi-million-dollar deal to train a police force. American health-care corporation Abt Associates, Inc., described as 'one of the largest for-profit government and business research and consulting firms in the world', was awarded a $44 million contract for the restructuring of Iraq's health-care system. Science Applications International Corporation (overseen by the US Defence Department's Office of Psychological Operations) received $100 million to take over the unsuccessful CPA-launched television station, though within a couple of months the corporation was being investigated for profiteering.

'These are not companies, they are gangsters,' announced Dr Sadek, my cynical colleague at the Ministry of Health. He pointed out a report in one of the new Baghdad papers about Bechtel's history of buying and privatising state water companies in developing countries, then increasing tariffs so that water became a commodity out of reach of the poor. Sadek declared that this second Gulf War had been the First War of Globalisation, aimed at forcing open Iraq's markets – and later those of Syria, Iran and the rest of the Middle East – with a thoroughness that the World Trade Organisation forums could never achieve. 'With the bombs and the looting they destroy everything; telephones, water, sanitation, our education, our medical service,' he snarled. 'Now they build it again, privatised, and make us pay to use it. They even appoint a new government to approve this robbery. You will see' – he lifted a prophetic finger – 'the people will not accept this.'

✚

We continued our work with the Ministry of Health doctors, distributing emergency drugs, treating where we could. Many Baghdad hospitals remained disaster areas. Besides the usual patients attending the city's emergency departments – heart attacks, diabetes, asthma exacerbated by the smoke of burning buildings – wounded citizens would arrive in numbers that the staff struggled to deal with. Those hit by bullets were usually young men, while children suffered injuries from the military ordnance that littered the city. I saw some kids brought in who'd found a cluster bomblet: one was dead, another deaf, his ear-drums ruptured by the blast, one foot mangled to a flap of skin like an empty sock. I helped to treat the victims after a grenade was tossed into a gasoline queue, causing an inferno of exploding jerrycans. Car after car pulled up, disgorging trembling casualties with blackened faces, clothing fused to their skin. We slathered Flamazine over the blisters, wrapping them in gauze. One man required an intravenous infusion to replace the fluid oozing from his burns. The only drip-site in undamaged skin was on the inside of his ankle. Despite the lack of local anaesthetic he lay still while I cut down to locate the vein, into which I slipped a plastic cannula that I stitched in place. The drip was connected and, along with his burns, covered and dressed. By now the man's family had arrived, and the nurses delivered him to their care with bags of intravenous fluid and dressings; treatment at home would be safer than on the unclean wards.

Each day, after clinics and hospitals and the afternoon CMCC briefings, the members of our medical group would meet at the hotel and take turns to enter data, field-reports and funding proposals to headquarters on our computers. The hotel pool had been filled with turbid Tigris water that soon cleared, and after work was done there was no greater pleasure I knew of in the city than to dive into the silky water and stroke my way through languorous lengths. One hot night, drying myself amidst the bubble-gum smell of the gardenias, I was invited to join a gathering that was drinking vodka at an adjacent table. The party consisted of an American documentary maker and some women war correspondents, grouped around a big, tough US Special Forces colonel who'd been appointed by the Pentagon as military liaison officer to Chalabi. The women all appeared greatly impressed by Chalabi's leadership qualities. The colonel they worshipped, describing in thrilled tones how he had taken from its plinth in the Republican Palace garden a bust of Saddam and replaced it with the head of a goat. The colonel knocked back his drink and demonstrated how he had sliced through the goat's neck with his belt knife in order to disarticulate the spine.

'The doc will know this,' he drawled, to gasps of awe. 'It's gettin' through the skin's the toughest part.'

The colonel was accustomed to lead, and he treated their attention as no more than his due. He was even something of an officer-philosopher, discoursing as he drank on the origins of the soldier's expression 'to get nicked'; derived, he claimed, not via the British army slang for being caught by the police, but from the passive form of the Arabic verb *niqa*, to fuck, so a comrade who 'got nicked' had been killed or critically injured. One of the women was tall and blond, with a sharp-faced attractiveness, and the vodka led her, via expressions of the really sincere love that she felt for every person present, into a broadcast of her intimate circumstances – 'I gotta million bucks' – and her patriotism: 'I was trained by the FBI you know that Colonel, but I stopped because you know you just can't trust them to protect you [eyelash flutter, slip into confidential huskiness], but I still work for them as a messenger and the CIA as well, Colonel.'

'Ah believe in livin' out in the open,' growled the colonel from his barrel chest. 'Let yur enemy come to you, then kill him.'

I excused myself from the party and went to change, then up to the roof to put a call in to my landlady. She agreed to a limited extension of her notice period so that I could 'hurry up and finish my work'. It was impossible to explain that our work was effectively unfinishable – the deteriorating conditions in Baghdad were undoing it all around us – and I wondered how soon, if I wasn't back by the new deadline, she'd dump my possessions on the street. I decided to visit some journalist friends on their hotel terrace. They poured me a stiff drink, while below us the women threw themselves into the pool with their clothes on.

'Oh, Colonel, Colonel!' their voices trilled amidst splashes and whoops. 'Look at me, Colonel!'

To the west, magnesium parachute-flares descended over a position being attacked in the suburbs and cannon-fire arced above the rooftops. As we watched, a mysterious transformation began to creep across the city. The acetylene-bright flares dimmed to a ghostly glimmer and the headlights of cars in the streets seemed suddenly to be illuminating tunnels of brown mist. Within a few minutes we were wrapped in an enervating heat, our eyes stinging as the sandstorm rolled over us. The drum-fire beyond the compound wall rose to a crescendo, drowning out the voices of the poolside party.

✛

Sand hung thick in the air as we set off the next morning for Ar-Ramadi, where I was to assess the children's hospital. We had been warned by the CMCC of the risks in going to the region. Falluja, halfway between Baghdad and Ar-Ramadi, was a no-go area; ever since the Americans had killed seventeen citizens who were demonstrating against their presence in the town, they had suffered repeated casualties in insurgent attacks. Ar-Ramadi was considered a den of subversives and we'd been advised to keep the windows closed, doors locked and seatbelts on at all times to prevent us from being dragged bodily from our vehicle. But like much official information in Baghdad, this had to be weighed against the word-of-mouth story, which suggested that the towns were at the moment reasonably safe for those who had no connection with the CPA.

'Here in the Sunni areas the resistance is political, not religious,' explained our translator, a sharp-thinking young man with a business degree who wanted to be rich only slightly less than he wanted the Americans out of his country. 'The Islamists might attack any Westerner, but they do not operate here.'

Reassured, I watched the desert pass by. The translator lit a cigarette.

'They also say that Saddam Hussein is hiding in Ar-Ramadi.'

The dust-pall wiped away the horizon all around, so that the highway on which we travelled seemed to bisect the floor of an unchanging brown bowl. Now and then the outlines of burned-out trucks rose out of the murk and fell behind. Convoys of US military fuel tankers loomed up ahead twenty to a string, the wind of their passage buffeting our vehicle with the monotony of a pulse. Each time the driver would hiss softly between his teeth and correct his alignment with a twitch of the wheel. Conversation had stopped as he concentrated on his work. My ears felt blocked from the waves of air pressure. I thought about the inadvisability of being on this most ambushed road in the country, in the midst of hurtling American gasoline tankers. They kept coming, their headlights glowing, our vehicle thrust sideways and rocking back, and I felt in the grip of a pervading unreality, as though there were no destination for this mesmeric, blind rush. Despite my fear, I fell asleep.

Sunlight woke me as we emerged from the mist and turned into Ar-Ramadi through a grove of palms. The streets were quiet and orderly after the crazed traffic of Baghdad, the fire-station, schools and administrative offices open and working. There were none of the ruins that we were so accustomed to in the capital, apart from the Ba'ath Party building and headquarters of the Mukhabarat secret police, which had been scientifically demolished. Indeed Saddam Hussein would never have chosen to hide out here; the people in this Sunni region had fought the British in the 1920s, they'd resisted Saddam's rule and now they were fighting the Americans for their freedom. The Euphrates ran through the town, fast and clear with sapphire depths. On its bank stood one of Saddam's palaces, now the local US military headquarters. The dictator's unpopularity here had been such that he'd found it necessary to have the side of the bridge facing the palace screened off with metal sheeting, so that the populace could not take pot-shots at his house. The Americans kept the screens, to block aiming points for RPGs. Black-painted Humvees, belonging to US intelligence operatives or security contractors, were parked in the courtyard of the town's police station.

The health directorate, clinics and paediatric hospital were undamaged and fully staffed, though in dire need of materials that had not been supplied since the start of the war. The doctors took me around the hospital, pointing out incubators without oxygen, the skinny babies on drips for gastro-enteritis. There was much resentment at the behaviour of the US detachment stationed at the hospital gates. The day before, the hospital director had complained to the town's military commander that his soldiers were violating social custom by trying to chat up the women entering the building. That evening the unit had been abruptly withdrawn; a few hours later looters arrived and stole the fuel for the emergency generator, with the hospital guards, disarmed by the Americans, unable to intervene. Beneath the impression of order, said one doctor, the town simmered. There were frequent army raids on homes. The American soldiers were accompanied by 'special police' – ex-Mukhabarat men previously associated with the worst repressions of the old regime – and hooded informers. As patrols drove by, people looked away and spat.

On the road into Falluja we passed a US checkpoint that had been raked with rockets the night before. The soldiers manning it watched from inside their armoured vehicles, only their heads showing through the hatches. The traffic ignored them; some of the hauliers, racing their horse-carts like chariots, spat graphic insults that the Americans could not understand, though they greatly amused the Iraqi members of our team. Relaxed by the sight of a town where the occupiers were being forced to lower their profile, our driver and translator proposed a meal at a favourite restaurant on Falluja's main street. We were welcomed inside and directed towards a table. The ornate tiled fountain in the middle of the room was dry, but water was poured from a bucket onto our hands. *Keffiyeh*-swathed men ate, drank tea, smoked *nargilh*. Those whose eyes I caught nodded courteously. We ate with our hands while about us the conversation swirled. I looked around at this foreign place, its contrast of dignity and violence, and realised that this was what I travelled for; to be lost within this incomprehensible communion.

Back in Baghdad that evening, sitting in the NGO Co-ordinating Committee meeting, the wonder of that insight would not leave me. The topic of the meeting was the ethics of protection for aid workers. There had been a spate of aid vehicle hijackings and pillage of warehouses. Now some organisations wanted armed watchmen to guard their compounds, while others objected that it would increase the vulnerability of those who refused to be associated with guns. I watched the familiar confrontations: the microtome rationality of the Frenchman, the Serb's portentousness, the dramatic declarations of principle. Outside, gunfire erupted. The newcomers exchanged excited glances but we could tell it was at least a block away. I reflected how completely my nervous system was merged into Baghdad's mesh of sounds and stimuli, the strum of adrenalin, the prescience of trouble round the corner. I wondered how I'd find my way home.

11

Remission

My parents live quietly now, in a village north of New York City on the edge of Long Island Sound. The old wooden house, with its honey coloured floorboards, is a place of warmth and comfort, full of books and the art and artefacts of a dozen countries collected in our family's travels. Dinner table conversations are intimate, meditative, sometimes touched by sadness at the fleeting nature of life, for many of their friends and colleagues, comrades and contemporaries, are gone or dying, with their extra-ordinary lives of people lost and reunited and surviving amidst the turmoil of war. We seldom speak of 'home', we are less expatriate than extemporate, wry exiles from a time when ideas like truth and freedom had different meanings. The neighbourhood hums with the sound of summer lawn mowers and the roaring autumn gales from leaf blowers, the scrape as shovels clear the pavement of winter snow. The residences along the shore are old second homes of granite or clapboard and great summer mansions with flagpoles and boathouses, and the sea rubs restlessly against the rocks. There are no flamingos, no surfers, but in warm weather as we breakfast in the garden at the table under the trees it is as though we were back at our old house in Durban, except that squirrels instead of monkeys scamper along the garage roof.

My mother gave up being a pathologist years ago; she paints. My father retired in stages from his orthopaedic professorship. At seventy he stopped operating but continued for another five years to scrub for surgery and assist the residents-in-training, handing on the surgical skills he'd learned through hard experience. Thereafter he carried on teaching and consulting and interpreting the obscure X-rays that would be brought to him to settle diagnostic disputes. He'd recently written the chapter on tuberculosis of the spine for a definitive American reference work on orthopaedic surgery. I was at the retirement party where he celebrated his decision to take a break.

Among the guests were many of his work colleagues, including the American surgeon who had first invited him to take up the post at the New York medical school a quarter of a century before. The man described their first meeting at the Hadassah Hospital in Jerusalem during the 1973 war, when they'd both gone to work as volunteer surgeons treating the many Israeli orthopaedic and trauma casualties.

'I was operating on a young soldier,' the American told me, 'trying to remove a bit of shrapnel embedded in his median nerve. The edges of the metal were jagged, like fishhooks, and I was frightened of damaging the nerve further and leaving him with a useless arm. This other guy who was working on the patient – we had lots of wounded and we were working hard and you didn't have time to meet all the other surgeons – this other guy, he picked up a knife. "It's easiest to split the fibres longitudinally", he said, "by slicing the neural sheath. Let me show you", and he did it with absolute precision, separating the nerve into two trunks without cutting any fibres, and leaving the fragment lying in the middle. That guy was your dad. I've been learning from him ever since.'

My father had instructed me as a medical student in the art of examination. The first stage of assessment was always visual. 'Observe', he'd taught, 'don't just look', and would enumerate the causes of asymmetry: swelling, wasting, spasm and deformity. It was only after watching the patient's own movements that he placed his hands on a joint and began the physical examination. I'd marvel at how his fingers, like those of a safe-cracker, picked up the slightest crepitation, the subtle jump of roughness as joints travelled through their arc of movement, the creak of arthritis, the clunk cause by bony block and the drag of contacted ligaments. At the same time he would watch the patient's face, alert for the tensed look that indicated the fear of impending pain; the so-called 'apprehension test' of a dislocating shoulder or patella.

I have shared his dismay at the lapsing of diagnostic expertise as clinical skills have become replaced by high-tech investigations. We'd both experienced the scenario of doctors, their backs to the unexamined patient, addressing their treatment decisions to the scan on the screen, and we chuckled together at the prescience of a cartoon that showed a white-coated clinician standing at a bedside, X-ray picture raised. 'You had a broken leg', he is explaining to the bemused patient, 'but we fixed it with Photoshop'.

In a cupboard upstairs lie the rolled degrees and certificates of my father's surgical and orthopaedic qualifications, among them the red-sealed scroll that proclaims him a Fellow of the Royal College of Surgeons. Another parchment attests his Hunterian Professorship, a rare academic distinction awarded by the College for his work on the surgical treatment of spinal tuberculosis. Fine print at the bottom requests the return of these documents to the Royal College of Surgeons on each Fellow's death. This is a task I will perform for him, and perhaps someone will eventually do the same for me. In our different fields we have been practitioners of the same crude art – that of cutting people open – but surgery is also a symphony of delicate manipulation and subtle chords; my father once showed me a scientific paper on the actions of the wing-muscles that control the flight of birds, comparing these to the microscopically adjusting, precision movements of a surgeon's hands.

The backs of his now are bruised and purple-marked, from collisions with door-frames and shelves, while lost in thought. I've inherited from him a similar clumsiness when abstracted, and an ability to focus my fingers, when I need to, for the job of cutting. He has also passed on to me his magnifying operating glasses, worn on the forehead and flipped down when needed – I expect to be using them more and more for fine work – and a few old surgical instruments kept by him for nostalgic reasons: a spreader for opening bullet tracks, a suture-needle holder he'd had made to his own design, a mahogany-cased British army field surgical kit with its amputation knives, bone saw, silver tracheotomy tubes and circular cutters to drill out discs of skull, each item stamped with the War Department's cipher. There is an osteotome for scraping the adherent membrane from bone, made in Solingen, Germany: part of the pannier of German army medical supplies captured in 1943 that had yielded up the Atabrin tablets he'd taken to Palestine. Every relic carries a story, part of the legacy of knowledge that has formed me as a person and a doctor. A file contains accounts of his adventurous times treating battle casualties in the Second World War and two Israeli conflicts, which he always said he'd turn into a book, but the outline typed up thirty years ago is yellowed, its corner marked from a paper clip corroded by Durban's soft rust.

Perhaps my father feels his stories have served their purpose, like the old instruments. I asked him recently to recount a story that had always entertained me, about the blood transfusion facility he and his colleagues had set up in 1948 at Israel's Military Hospital Number Ten for resuscitation of the wounded. When an offensive was due, bottled blood, pre-typed, would be readied in the receiving area. As casualties arrived from the battlefield the surgeons would assess the degree of shock, check the patient's type from his ID tag and call for blood, which would be hooked onto an overhead wire and shunted along to the bay for immediate transfusion. Once, when everyone had their hands full dealing with injured that filled the casualty bays, the hospital's officious CO appeared and started shouting orders and getting underfoot. Told by one of the doctors to shut up and make himself useful, he'd sent the wrong blood-bottle along the wire, causing the patient a violent haemolytic reaction and subsequent kidney failure. It had turned out that the commanding officer knew nothing of blood typing but was acquainted with an anaesthetist who had made a dialysis machine from a description he'd read in a science magazine; they'd used it until the man's kidneys recovered, and saved his life.

My dad smiled at my promptings.

'It's true. It happened', was all he said. And then a bit later: 'You know, in those days we practiced heroic medicine. The heroes were the patients'.

We discuss advances in the treatment of war casualties. Lifesaving techniques are most effective in the first hour after injury, before shock and infection have set in. Soldiers carry new dressing bandages impregnated with compounds that encourage blood-clotting, to stop haemorrhage. A specialised dressing – the Asherman Chest Seal, designed to cover sucking chest wounds while acting as a one-way valve to re-inflate the collapsed lung – will go into medical kits. A super-antibiotic is being researched for administration to every casualty at the earliest moment, and synthesised blood solutions are in development for emergency transfusion. In 1989 I'd worked on one of the preliminary projects testing synthetic blood, at an American university hospital. Alongside my master's degree research on the treatment of arterial disease, I had been part of a team carrying out experimental infusions of a formulation of haemoglobin – the oxygen-carrying compound normally sealed inside red blood cells – structurally modified to prevent the free molecule causing damage to kidney and lung.

Two years later, in 1991, I was working as a surgeon in northern Iraq. Casualties sometimes reached me in shock from blood loss. Transfusion was needed for resuscitation and effective surgery, but our hospital consisted of two tents in a meadow with a stretcher set up outside as an operating table to take advantage of the daylight. There was no electricity and no refrigeration for blood, even if we'd had the means of obtaining and cross-matching it, and patients died who might otherwise have been saved. A synthesised haemoglobin solution can be mass-produced, stored on a shelf and given to anyone. In trials, large amounts of the compound have been infused into trauma cases suffering massive haemorrhage – enough to replace the patient's blood volume twice over – without problematic side-effects. My father and I talk about how we could both have done with having this stuff available in the field.

But planned advances are even more imaginative. The US Army is working on technology to monitor the physiological status of each soldier through sensors embedded in their uniforms. A global positioning system, combined with readouts of pulse rate, temperature and blood oxygen levels, will allow the battlefield medic to identify the location of a wounded soldier and the degree of injury, allowing the most serious casualties to be attended first. Military trauma-care planners envision the process becoming automated, with each casualty being laid in a 'critical care module' that will provide intensive monitoring of vital signs and give intravenous fluid and medication; some propose the development of 'remote telepresence surgery vehicles' in which emergency surgery can be performed by a surgeon based at a distant Mobile Advanced Surgical Hospital (MASH) using robotically manipulated surgical instruments to control bleeding, repair damaged tissue and stitch wounds.

My father and I – accustomed to one-way chest valves made from a bottle and a bit of tubing, improvising Tobruk-type splints for compound fractures – exchange cynical smiles. Roughly one in five of the world's nations are currently involved in wars or insurgencies or armed unrest, the vast majority the sort of technologically crude conflicts I had witnessed in Mozambique, Burma, Angola and Eritrea. The care I'd been able to provide for those wounded had been basic; even in Baghdad, where some patients had been injured by the world's most advanced weaponry, there was no commensurate sophistication in the treatment available. For these and other largely civilian victims of this global bloodshed, computerised advances in operative surgery and even Asherman seals seem a remote way off. Essential trauma management – casualty assessment, resuscitation and emergency surgery – will be the main line of treatment in most parts of the world for the foreseeable future. Surgeons will need to know how to use their hands to assess a wounded patient and to expose major blood vessels, open a chest or get into an abdomen in a hurry.

American computer experts are designing digital casualties to provide their military surgeons with a sort of dry run for the real thing, but despite extraordinary advances in stereoscopic imaging, 'force-feedback' controls and Total Immersion Virtual Reality simulation, it is uncertain if this electronic training can prepare a surgeon to deal with the incalculable shock of real war and death. I recall a conversation I had with my father the last time he was mobilised for the treatment of major casualties, shortly before he retired. In September 2001 I'd been back from Angola for a couple of months and was more or less readjusted to peacetime life – sitting in a coffee shop – when the news came that the New York World Trade Centre towers had been struck by hijacked aircraft. I called my father at his hospital to find out whether he'd made contact with the rest of the family: my sister and mother, due to be in the air that day flying back to New York, and my brother working in downtown Manhattan. Having established that everyone was accounted for, I asked what was happening at the hospital.

'Disbelief', he said. 'The first tower was burning in the distance as I drove to work, and it looked so strange that I couldn't work out what it was. By the time I reached my consulting room the second tower was hit. There was an announcement that the hospital's major disaster plan was being activated, and we went down into the Civil Defence basement under the emergency department and brought out a couple of hundred gurneys and lined them up in the street with pillows and blankets and intravenous fluid bags hanging on the drip stands. That was two hours ago. We haven't received a single casualty and now with the collapse of the towers we aren't going to. The doctors have set up television sets in the street. They're standing out there in their surgical greens and they're watching the broadcasts and looking at the smoke, and they're crying'.

Nothing in the training of these young doctors had prepared them for the experience of seeing a catastrophe unfold and being unable to do anything about it. I could imagine their shock and helplessness. I had learned, like my father, the limitations of our craft; sometimes there's nothing you can do to help. But you keep going, and the next time, maybe, you can.

☩

These are things for which we have to be prepared, for an age of uncertainty is upon us, with continuing attacks on our cities amidst an endless war that will blur the distinction between military and civilian medical practice. The medical services of American and British armed forces, already committed in Afghanistan, were only able to meet the shortfall in surgeons during the second Gulf War and consequent Iraqi insurgency by an extended call-up of reservists from civilian hospitals. With the 2004 train bombs in Madrid, hospitals received the less critically injured casualties first and began treating them; when those arrived needing life-saving emergency surgery, doctors and operating theatres were already occupied. It is difficult for surgeons in their normal practice to develop competence in the demanding field of intensive trauma care, especially with the increasing trend in doctors' training towards narrow specialisation.

I had never imagined that my misspent professional career, with its squandered opportunities for advancement, could qualify as any sort of expertise. But it seems that this experience in marginal areas of medicine has acquired an acute relevance. I am asked to address medical groups on humanitarian surgery work, or to talk about operating in the 'austere environment' – under battlefield conditions – to military doctors. In London, the august medical examining body called the Worshipful Society of Apothecaries (its royal charter dating from 1617) has just inaugurated a new, dedicated Faculty of Conflict and Catastrophe Medicine; to my surprise, I have been included among those practitioners whom, 'in view of [their] interest and expertise in this area', have been invited to become members of Faculty. My haphazard occupation has become a specialty.

Periodically I serve as a tutor on courses designed to prepare surgeons for future conflict. Held at the Royal College of Surgeons in London and the medical faculty of the University of Nijmegen in Holland, they teach the management of major trauma. Within these esteemed institutions I cannot help but feel an impostor, for it seems improbable that my war-zone assignments – unpredictable, often chaotic – can qualify me in any way to advise experienced colleagues and trained young surgeons in trauma care. But I realise that my work in places like Eritrea and Kurdistan has taught me rare lessons about dealing with mass casualties, assessing swiftly each patient's condition and injuries for assignment to treatment priorities. This is a brutal science demanding a dispassion seldom called upon in normal clinical situations, for as a result of these decisions some wounded will receive attention and others will be left to die. It combines broad considerations – surgical, anaesthetic and nursing facilities available, the accessibility of blood transfusion and evacuation – with specific knowledge about which injuries kill quickest, for this dictates the order in which treatment is applied. At its simplest, patients with life-threatening wounds that can be treated rapidly with a good likelihood of survival will fall into the most urgent priority, followed by those who have severe injuries but can be stabilised to wait their turn, and finally the non-urgent who can tolerate long delays. There is a fourth group whose categorisation is 'expectant'; those with massive injuries that will require intensive treatment exceeding available resources, and who are therefore placed aside for later reassessment when time and facilities become available, should they still be alive.

The theory of triage surgery can be taught in a book. Its practice requires being able to treat the immediate-priority injuries that threaten rapid death – clinical situations in which the only medical information may be the mark of an entrance wound and the account that signs of life had been present in the past few minutes – and these require a lightning surgical approach. I've experienced how easy it is to get it wrong. A third of gunshot wounds to the mid-chest will require abdominal surgery too, and in up to forty percent of major trauma operations the first incision will be into the wrong space; an art lies in realising that the patient's dropping blood pressure and deepening shock is not explained by the visible injuries and that another source for the collapse must be found, by a rapid extension of the search into areas – neck, pelvis, the back of the abdomen – that might be outside one's familiar operating territory.

The shock of the July 2005 bombings in London has galvanised awareness of this sort of training, for few civilian surgeons will have had to deal with the complex blast and fragmentation injuries of military-style trauma; even military surgeons traditionally were left to re-learn such skills by trial and error on the wounded of the next war. These surgery courses teach you how. They are taught on the closest alternative to living people: dead ones. Bodies, bequeathed by their owners to the advancement of medical knowledge, are training trauma surgeons in the preservation of life. The course participants learn precisely what's involved in cutting through the ribcage to get into chests, to stitch wounds in the heart or lacerated lung. They open the belly, working fast and systematically as they'll do on a real casualty, checking the quadrants of the abdomen for bleeding, packing haemorrhage sites, mobilising the liver to explore the deep vessels behind.

The shattering wounds and death and mortal terror that I have seen in wars in remote parts of the world have come among us. These young surgeons, instruments in hand, concentrate on ways to confront their enemy. Under the operating lights a soft mist rises from the exposed tissue. As I lean between the shoulders of the tutorial group clustered around a dissection table, in order to demonstrate a point of surgical access, something caresses my hip: a hand, pale and waxen. I look down at the face, hollowed back to bare anatomy, and know at once our brotherhood.

❖

I think of my long familiarity with death: the living who struggled to survive and the children who did not fight but renounced life unquestioningly. I have become conditioned to loss and uncertainty. Yet this journey, far exceeding my youthful imaginings, has made me oddly adapted to the world's new requirements. The fairy tales are right to warn that you should be very, very careful what you wish for. I travel in the sorts of places I'd dreamed about, embrace the sorts of causes, and though I was never much good at Liar Dice, I've continued drawing heavily on my luck. My father has always known how little he could say to prepare his son for that first step into risk, for the Art is long and Experience fallacious, and the really vital things cannot be taught. I remember his advice, shortly before I departed for my first war, when I'd asked him for the essential knowledge he'd discovered in his journeying that I would need to know in order to survive.

'Well, there are two things, really'. He had looked at me, smiling. 'Never miss an opportunity of filling your stomach, or emptying your bladder'.

Our family continues to travel between America and South Africa and points between, dodging the winter where possible. Now and then we gather for a fortnight among the cypresses of a hilltop farm in northern Italy, belonging to the daughter of a man to whom my grandfather had exported fine leather from South Africa between the wars. At our most recent reunion we sat together watching old home movies: my parents' honeymoon in the Belgian Congo; a stay on the Italian Riviera when my brother and I were toddlers; beach holidays in the Cape. Suddenly I found myself looking at a piece of film that I had last seen in the 1960s. It is about twelve minutes long, in saturated blues and browns, shot at a sanatorium outside Durban as a presentation on the treatment of spinal tuberculosis for an international orthopaedic conference.

The camerawork is my mother's, as are the hand-painted intertitles. My father, in white trousers and safari jacket, chats without sound to a Zulu child of about ten; her mother, in tribal beadwork, looks on anxiously. He sits the girl forward and we see the humped deformity of her back where the disease has collapsed the vertebrae. They walk together, her gait stiff and jerky from the pressure on the nerves. Then there is the surgery, the blood rich as rubies, the delicate dissection as carious bone is whittled out from against the spinal cord. On the operating table the angulated back is slowly straightened. The clean cavity of the missing vertebrae yawns and a graft of rib-bone, precisely shaped, slots into the gap. In the next scene, three months later, the girl walks erect, her stride flowing. There is joy on her face. My mother's steady hand on the camera frames my tall, smiling father, the child made straight: the absolute clarity of good vanquishing ill.

✛

I wish I might somehow rediscover that clear resolution in my own work. It used to be, before we went into Iraq in 2003, that there were assumptions that could be made about the worth – and the price – of voluntary doctoring in conflict zones. We believed the benefits outweighed the dangers, for aid workers were not generally sought out as targets by the people they came to help. The global battle-lines that the war engendered changed all that. Soon suicide bombers would target the UN's Baghdad headquarters and the offices of the International Red Cross, and by the end of the year even the most dedicated aid agencies, with decades of selfless work in Iraq, would find it impossible to continue operating as their personnel became targets for abduction and murder.

Among the many casualties of that war has been the idealism we offered. Now some of the Iraqi doctors and international humanitarian workers who were my colleagues are dead, while the private security contractors thrive, charging up to ten thousand dollars for the seven-mile transfer between Baghdad airport and the city centre. Humanitarian intervention is changed, perhaps forever; along with it the justification for what has given meaning to a large part of my life. Perhaps it is time for me to renounce those dreams, to settle down, to think of having children of my own to whom I can pass on my own relics: a worn copy of *A Simple Guide to Trauma* with the bitter dust of crushed malaria tablets between its pages; an Ethiopian shell-fragment that gouged the earth beside me on the Zalambessa front; the compact canvas pouch of surgical instruments I've carried since my first war in Kurdistan. But every day I read the war news like job-vacancy ads, looking for peace.

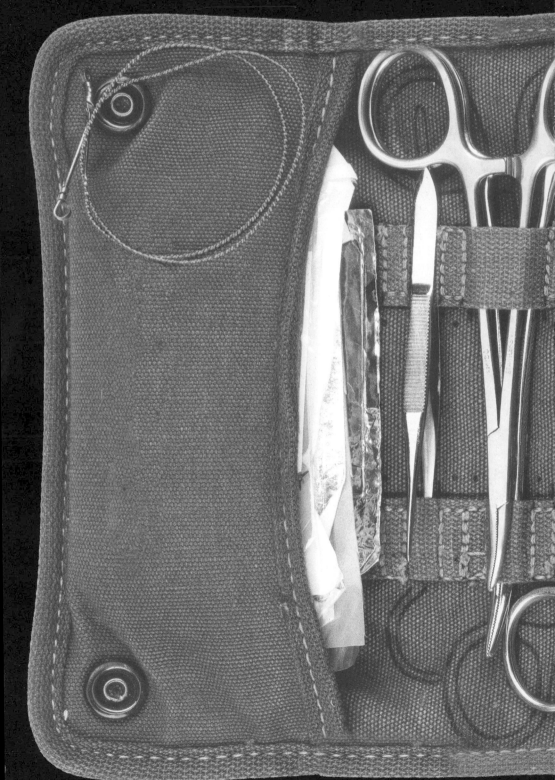